TABLE OF CONTENTS

Plenary Session I
Nature and Magnitude of the Problem

Plenary Session II
Specific Aspects of the Problem

Plenary Session III
Social Policy and Service Aspects of the Problem

Plenary Session IV
Reports of Discussion Groups

BATTERED CHILDREN
AND CHILD ABUSE

ok is to be retur

Proceedings of the XIXth CIOMS Round Table Confe ace

Berne, Switzerland
4–6 December 1985
Edited by Z. Bankowski and M. Carballo

A07102

Organized jointly by the
Council for International Organizations of Medical Sciences
and the
World Health Organization

Acknowledgements

The Council for International Organizations of Medical Sciences (CIOMS) and the World Health Organization (WHO) wish to express their gratitude to all individuals, organizations and institutions for their help and contributions, which made this conference possible.

We are particularly grateful to Professor M.C. Bettex, President of the World Federation of Associations of Paediatric Surgeons and Director of the University Children's Clinic, Berne, upon whose initiative this conference became a reality, and to his colleagues, Drs B. Kehrer and T. Slongo, who ensured that the conference was run smoothly and in a most pleasant atmosphere.

We express special thanks to the Max and Elsa Beer-Brawand Fund, the Swiss Academy of Medical Sciences, the Swiss National Fund and Migros Enterprise for substantial financial support.

Thanks are also extended to Dr J. Gallagher for his assistance in editing the proceedings of the conference.

Programme and Organizing Committee

Bankowski, Z. Council for International Organizations of Medical Sciences, Geneva

Belsey, M.A. Unit of Maternal and Child Health, World Health Organization, Geneva

Bettex, M.C. Chirurgische Universitäts-Kinderklinik, Berne; World Federation of Associations of Paediatric Surgeons; Chairman, Conference Organizing Committee, Berne

Carballo, M. Unit of Maternal and Child Health, World Health Organization, Geneva

Kehrer, B. Department of Paediatric Surgery, Universitäts-Kinderklinik, Berne

Orley, J. Division of Mental Health, World Health Organization, Geneva

Petros-Barvazian, A. Division of Family Health, World Health Organization, Geneva

Shah, P.M. Unit of Maternal and Child Health, World Health Organization, Geneva

Slongo, T. Department of Paediatric Surgery, Universitäts-Kinderklinik, Berne

Preface

Conferences of the Council for International Organizations of Medical Sciences (CIOMS) are interdisciplinary forums which enable scientists and lay people to express their views on topics of immediate concern, unhampered by administrative, political or other considerations. They are designed not only to present the scientific and technical basis of new developments in biology and medicine but also to explore their social, ethical, moral, administrative, economic and legal implications.

Participants in these conferences include prominent representatives of the fields of medicine and biology, philosophy and theology, sociology and law; it is felt that this multidisciplinary approach can best increase understanding of issues that are no longer exclusively the concern of any one profession and are sometimes the subject of wide public interest.

Child battering and child abuse in general is becoming widespread, possibly differing in the forms it takes from one cultural setting to another but always with medical, social, legal and ethical implications. This conference, organized jointly with the Division of Family Health of the World Health Organization (WHO), was designed as an interdisciplinary international forum for discussion and reflection on how the problem should be taken up by national and international bodies.

The need for a conference on this subject reflects a growing public awareness and concern about the problem of child abuse in both developed and developing countries. This concern has been stimulated by the dramatic increase observed in recent years in the number of reported cases of child abuse, as well as by a better understanding among the public and professionals of the many different forms that child abuse takes in different social and economic settings. Although the reported increase has been particularly noticeable in the industrialized countries, it is believed that the problem is by no means restricted to these countries and that in what are predominantly traditional, rural and agricultural societies child abuse may be equally extensive, albeit not as well diagnosed or reported.

Z. Bankowski
Executive Secretary, CIOMS

INTRODUCTION

M. Carballo

World Health Organization, Geneva

Nature of the Problem—Like the realization that children have special needs and hence special rights, the discovery of child abuse as a global problem has had to await the second half of the twentieth century. The problem, however, is not new. There is considerable historical evidence that prior to the European industrial revolution, and certainly during it, systematic maltreatment of children for both economic and ideological reasons was common. At various times, growing awareness of the problem as it affected disadvantaged groups led to calls for social reform and policies designed to protect the health and well-being of children, especially during periods of social disruption. It was not until the second half of this century, however, that any widespread attempt was made to seek an explanation of the problem or, what is more important, ways of systematically controlling and preventing it as well as treating the victimized child.

Despite this attempt and the considerable attention the problem has received in recent years, child abuse remains a largely neglected policy area, one on which it has not been possible to obtain any widespread understanding or agreement as to the steps that can and should be taken to combat it. Few countries, for example, have seriously begun to monitor its incidence or to describe its magnitude. Even fewer have taken steps to formulate training programmes to train the different health and social staff who deal with abused children.

Magnitude of the Problem—It remains difficult to determine the true magnitude of the problem in most countries, developed or developing. The problem of inadequate data is not peculiar to any particularly country or region, but, as with other health indicators, it is much more serious in developing than in developed countries, where health information systems lend themselves more readily to the reporting of child abuse. Even where routine reporting is common, however, the quality of the available information remains variable. Incidence rates currently in use are drawn from a variety of sources: in some instances, national surveys and central reporting registers constitute reasonably reliable sources; in others it is still necessary to rely on compilations of newspaper accounts, or to calculate estimates by extrapolating from case studies or small surveys.

What data do exist nevertheless suggest that, as the public and health and social workers have become more aware of the problem and as monitoring systems have improved, estimates of incidence rates have been consistently revised upwards. Rates of between 13 and 21 per 1,000 population have been reported in industrialized countries. Hospital data on so-called accidental injuries that are also attributable to wilful abuse indicate that the problem may be equally serious in developing countries. The continued lack of legal requirements to report cases in many countries, however, makes it difficult to analyse trends reliably or to formulate or evaluate programmes to prevent or treat child abuse.

Moreover, most published data refer to individual cases of child battering and sexual abuse that have been brought before the courts or to hospitals. These are an important segment of the problem and call for immediate and specific action. However, they involve relatively very few children compared with the very much greater numbers associated with societal faults. There are, for instance, according to conservative estimates, 145 million children between the ages of 10 and 14 years involved in child labour, and chronic severe poverty in some parts of the world contributes to infant and young child mortality rates of 160 per 1,000 and of large-scale abandonment of children.

Definition—A fundamental constraint to monitoring, better comparative analysis, and realistic estimates of the magnitude of the problem is that definitions of child abuse vary both within and between countries. Even within countries the health, social welfare and legal sectors perceive the problem differently.

This lack of unanimity reflects differences in the technical approaches developed by the different professions concerned with child abuse, and their tendency to use terms that express their own ideas about the nature of the problem and what they can contribute to diagnosis and treatment.

Internationally, there have been equally limiting differences with regard to attitudes and traditions in child rearing and child disciplining; families and communities may see children as economic resources, and this complicates the difficulty of establishing definitions that are acceptable to different cultural groups.

Attempts to define and operationalize the concept, especially in the context of non-industrialized societies, have till recently also been hampered because much of the analytic work on child abuse has been based on studies from developed countries. Although child abuse has been shown to occur, in one form or another, in many non-industrialized, rural and traditional societies, most of them have not regarded it as a serious social problem, and consequently have taken no important social steps to deal with it or to establish a policy with regard to it.

With little agreement between the various disciplines and sectors concerned with the needs of children, and without a standardized international approach, it remains difficult not only to compare national trends and international rates but also to develop feasible and problem-specific ways of responding to and preventing child abuse.

For the purposes of the conference, the generic term "child abuse" was employed to refer to any intended or unintended act or omission by an adult, society or country, which adversely affects a child's health, physical growth or psychosocial development. The term is also meant to cover acts and omissions which the child may not necessarily regard as abusive or neglectful, and, conversely, behaviour of adults which they may not recognize as abusive.

It was nevertheless recognized that various other terms are in common use and that, in different settings, they serve to distinguish between different forms of child abuse. These terms include "maltreatment", which is sometimes used in an all-embracing way to refer not only to parental behaviour but also to actions (as well as omissions) of other individuals, groups, organizations, institutions or society at large which "jeopardise the physical, social, mental, or moral development of the child to some degree"[1]. Used in this sense, the term covers behaviour patterns which, whether sanctioned by law and custom or not, are in some way injurious to the child's health or social, economic, emotional or moral well-being.

Sometimes the term "child abuse" has been narrowly focused to refer only to parental acts that constitute a misuse or exploitation of the rights of parents and guardians with regard to the control and disciplining of the children under their care[2]. According to this usage, child abuse occurs when a parent or guardian knowingly misuses his privileged position vis-à-vis the child in order to commit acts which transgress societal norms and damage the child's development as a full and functioning member of society. It may be emotional or psychological abuse, harming the child's normal personality development; it is often characterized by "continual scapegoating, terrorizing and rejection"[3] of the child. "Sexual abuse" is usually defined as any sexual misuse of the child by a parent or guardian or other family-related adult. "Drug abuse" usually refers to deliberate drugging of children by adults with preparations intended for use by adults, or the sharing of narcotics and alcoholic drinks with them[4]. "Child battering", which differs from "physical abuse" only in degree or severity, is often used to describe acts that require medical attention and treatment, or that leave bruises on the child.

The concept of "child neglect", or "passive child abuse", usually refers to the failure by parents or guardians to perform duties and obligations which are basic to the child's well-being, such as supervision, nurture, protection, and the provision of food, clothing, medical care and education. "Child exploitation" refers to forms of child abuse from which the perpetrator gains economic benefits, and generally refers to the compelling of children to engage in paid employment in work or environments that harm their general physical psychosocial and moral development.

While these definitions are no doubt of analytic and reporting value, it was nevertheless felt that the more general term "child abuse" could adequately encompass these different variations and, at the same time, provide a sense of their impact on, and implications for, the victimized child. For the purpose of developing or promoting social policies, moreover, an all-inclusive term such as "child abuse" may have advantages.

Explanatory Models—A number of psychiatric, sociological, and ecological frameworks have been proposed to help explain the etiology of child abuse, and to permit the determination of ways in which the problem might be controlled and prevented. For a variety of methodological reasons, some of which have been referred to above, definitive conclusions concerning causal or precipitating factors are difficult to draw on the basis of some of these models.

Theoretical approaches to the problem have, in general, built on specific linear models of behaviour such as concern the psychopathologic or special child. While not without their value, linear models are limited with respect to their ability to accommodate such intervening phenomena as rapid social change, family disorganization and the impact of these changes on interpersonal relationships and behaviour. There is a recent trend to use a multivariate approach, in which reciprocal relationships between children, those who are immediately responsible for their care, the family unit and society can be viewed in a dynamic fashion.

Socioecological multivariate models are of use also in that they set child abuse

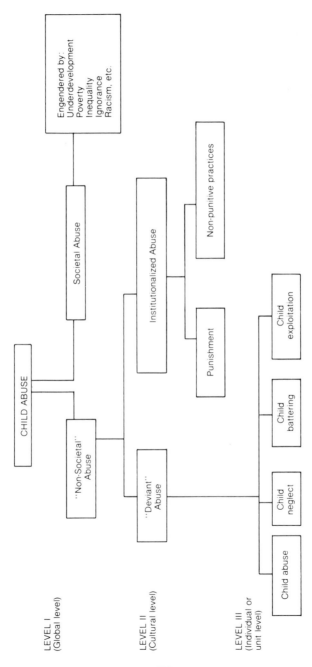

Figure 1: Child abuse: analytical model.

LEVEL I
(Global level)

LEVEL II
(Cultural level)

LEVEL III
(Individual or
unit level)

CHILD ABUSE

Societal Abuse

Engendered by:
Underdevelopment
Poverty
Inequality
Ignorance
Racism, etc.

"Non-Societal"
Abuse

Institutionalized Abuse

"Deviant"
Abuse

Punishment

Non-punitive practices

Child abuse

Child
neglect

Child
battering

Child
exploitation

IX

against a broad sociopolitical background; as a result, they indicate that the best way to understand and deal with child abuse may be by building a new socioecological system. In this regard, the framework outlined below, a modified version of the model presented by Obikeze at the conference[5], helps in the understanding of societal forms of child abuse and their relationship to other forms and their origins.

The model encompasses the general definitions presented above as well as the conference use of the term "child abuse". In introducing societal abuse, it highlights a problem which is not usually referred to in the clinical literature and not often represented in the analytical or explanatory models that have been proposed but which nevertheless may be the most pervasive and affect the health and welfare of the most children, particularly in developing countries.

The concept of societal child abuse refers to a global condition in which the lack of social, economic and other development resources affects adversely the growth and development of children. It refers specifically to societies where poverty, hunger, poor sanitation, inadequate shelter and lack of health care contribute to infant mortality rates that are at times as high as 160 per 1000. In parts of Asia, Africa and Latin America, children under the age of six years account for half of all deaths, or up to 80% of all children may be underweight, or 20% of all children die before their fifth birthday. Such data draw attention to an abuse of children that is fundamentally societal.

This concept includes also the abuse of children that is associated with chronic war, into which children are being increasingly drawn and in which very many are killed or exposed over long periods to abusive psychological stress. Similarly it refers to the poor access to education and the limited possibilities that many children have of developing their potential, which are increasingly common in large population groups in developing countries.

Extra-familial child abuse of this type is far more widespread than the intra-familial form; it tends to be hidden except in crises, and has yet received neither adequate attention from the public nor the serious concern of decision-makers. Child labour, child prostitution, chronic malnutrition and economic insecurity, as well as the submitting of children to the numbing brutality of war, are issues that merit immediate action, both nationally and internationally.

Extra-familial and intra-familial child abuse appear to have certain common causes and associations, such as poverty, social inequity, ignorance, racism and unemployment. Conditions of social tension, inequity and economic crisis are known to contribute directly and indirectly to both forms; it seems likely therefore that, although the true magnitude of child abuse is unknown, its present incidence will continue and even increase unless there is a decisive social and political commitment to broad social and specific coordinated action to deal with it.

Action to Deal with Child Abuse

Broad health and social strategies based on primary and secondary prevention of child abuse have recently been proposed. Primary prevention emphasizes the stimulation of interest in, and a better understanding of, the health and social aspects of child abuse; more responsible and informed parenthood and, by extension, support for the family; and a better allocation of social and institutional resources likely to support healthy family functioning. These are, by their nature, long-term measures, but any action taken to achieve them is likely to draw attention to the nature of child abuse, its magnitude, and its biological and psychosocial effects on the individual child and on children in general.

Secondary prevention, including the definition and recognition of individual, familial, and community risk characteristics and circumstances likely to be associated with, or to predispose to, child abuse, consists of direct short-term ways of reducing threats to children and improving conditions that place them at risk.

Prevention and therapy have focused on individual cases of battering and other forms of abuse. Given the reported incidence of child battering in certain highly industrialized countries, this is not surprising. As a result of the rediscovery in recent years of the battered child syndrome, and of improved guidelines for clinical diagnosis of child abuse, the numbers of reported cases have increased continuously. The publicity attached to these and other forms of intra-familial abuse, including sexual abuse, has increased awareness among health and social workers and led to more reporting by the public. Certainly in the United States, where the problem has received considerable attention from the media and in training programmes, recent data suggest that the incidence of some types of child abuse may have peaked and that preventive measures are beginning to reduce the number of new cases.

In general, action has been forthcoming from a variety of sectors including health, social welfare and the judiciary. Many organizations, both governmental and non-governmental, have by now accumulated experience and have perfected ways of dealing with specific aspects of the problem. What has been lacking, however, with the exception of a few countries and international efforts, has been the systematic compilation and analysis of these experiences so that they might be more widely disseminated and adapted to different cultural and social situations. Similarly, comprehensive national strategies or coordinated global efforts to mobilize technical and moral support for programmes in this area have largely been lacking.

In some countries, concern over the increase in abused and neglected children has led to an enactment of new laws. In some jurisdictions special laws have been introduced to deal with child abuse as part of criminal law; in others, meanwhile, the general criminal law applies and the legal protection of abused children is adequately covered by child protection acts and the civil courts. However, it cannot be too strongly emphasized that child abuse and neglect is not limited to intra-familial forms. In such forms as child prostitution, trafficking in children, forced marriage, exploitative and illegal labour, and generally degrading treatment it affects millions of children. New national legislation, and its enforcement, must take account of this. International Labour Organization (ILO) conventions have addressed many of these abuses and should be reflected more in domestic legislation. Education of the community with regard to the different forms that abuse takes, and to the existence and applicability of local laws, could result in better reporting and the early identification of children at risk.

Nevertheless, there is much more that non-governmental organizations, both professional and others, could do. Physicians, nurses, teachers, jurists and social workers, as well as religion-affiliated lay groups, trade unions, women and youth groups, and consumer and advocacy groups need to be encouraged to play a far more important role than they do at present, and more information will have to be made available to them. This could no doubt be accomplished more efficiently if there were specific and well-publicized national policies on the problem. At governmental level, ministries of health and social welfare, justice, labour, and education could also take on a more effective role if there were better coordinated policies on the prevention and treatment of child abuse. National research institutions and the media could equally, through ministerial programmes, contribute to educational activities designed to prevent and deal with the problem.

The management of "clinical" intra-familial child abuse has developed considerably in some countries but much remains to be done with regard to the early identification of high-risk circumstances, and the direct treatment and rehabilitation of the child, with the least disruption to the family, in which the child may have to continue to live. A managerial aspect often overlooked has been the counselling of families and providing them with the types of social support likely to improve parental functioning and child care in general.

As regards both intra- and extra-familial child abuse, political, legislative and regulatory action needs to be linked with improved monitoring systems; such linkage would, in turn, lead to situation-specific training programmes for health and social workers who are likely to be in a position to intervene.

In general, however, the principal need is for greater public awareness of the different forms of child abuse and the extent to which it occurs in different social circumstances. A variety of ways of informing and educating the public, and of training professional workers, are needed in order to ensure that child abuse receives adequate attention.

The conference, by consensus, adopted the following recommendations:

1. Since no well organized services can be provided in the absence of explicit policies and an allocation and acceptance of responsibility and since services for child abuse are lacking in many countries, and given that community organizations have a vital role to play in the early identification and prevention of child abuse, the Conference recommended that:

   governments designate national focal points with the responsibility of gathering information on the incidence of child abuse, compiling and disseminating technical documentation on the problem, providing advice and training materials, and advising all other national authorities on the subject.

2. Given the role that international agencies and organizations have played in promoting and coordinating actions for health and social welfare, and given their mandate with regard to the development of international instruments and standards relating to the promotion and protection of rights, the Conference recommended that:

   the World Health Organization and other agencies prepare a survey of policies, laws, and practices relating to the prevention and control of child abuse and neglect in selected developed and developing countries, in order to provide the type of evaluative framework that would permit other countries to develop or perfect approaches to the problem.

3. In view of the need for primary prevention of child abuse, including the sensitization of the public at large and the training of professional groups, and given the experience that has been gained in different countries, the Conference recommended that:

> steps be taken to set up coordinating mechanisms at an international level in order to provide a channel for the exchange of information between governmental and non-governmental agencies with a view to creating a better awareness of the problem and fostering progress in ways of dealing with it, at both the community and the professional levels.

4. Noting that the magnitude, as well as the impact, of child abuse, both intra- and extra-familial, are insufficiently well-known, and given that it will be difficult to develop appropriate policies and action in the absence of better epidemiological descriptions of the problem, the Conference recommended that:

> national and international groups and agencies carry out surveys of existing materials and reports, or undertake new surveys, in order to define the extent of the problem of child abuse, in its different forms, so as to provide a basis for policy and action.

5. Noting the close interrelationship between the social and the health aspects of child abuse, the need for promotional and technical activities designed to reach both the public and professional groups, and the need for coordination between international groups and agencies, the Conference recommended that:

> the World Health Organization establish a task force, representing different countries and disciplines, which could respond to requests for technical cooperation from countries, and could assist in the development of new policies based on updated analyses of the global situation, paying special attention to the long-term implications of child abuse for healthy growth and development.

References

[1] Veillard-Cybulska, H. The legal welfare of children in a disturbed family situation. *International Child Welfare Review,* No. 27, December 1975.
[2] Giovannoni, J.M. Parental mistreatment: Perpetrators and victims. *Journal of Marriage and Family,* Vol. 22, 1971.
[3] Schmitt, B.D. Battered child syndrome. In: *Current Pediatric Diagnosis and Treatment,* H.C. Kempe et al. (eds.) Los Altos, California, Lange Medical Publications, 1980.
[4] *ibid.*
[5] Obikeze, D.S. *Child maltreatment in non-industrialized countries: A framework for analysis.* Presented at the CIOMS/WHO Conference on Battered Children and Child Abuse, Berne, Switzerland, 4–6 December 1985.

OPENING ADDRESSES

M. Belchior

Council for International Organizations of Medical Sciences

It gives me much pleasure to welcome Dr Roos, Director of the Swiss Federal Office of Public Health. To be in your country, Dr Roos, is a great pleasure to the participants of this conference, and we are very appreciative of all your help. Dr Gellhorn, former President of CIOMS, professor of medicine, expert in medical education, New York State Department of Health: it is not easy, Dr Gellhorn, to thank you properly for everything you have done for CIOMS. Accepting the chairmanship of the conference at very short notice shows how much we can still ask of you and how much you can still do for us. Dr Petros-Barvazian, Director of the Division of Family Health of the World Health Organization: I do not think we could have this conference if we did not have your contribution and the assistance of your colleagues. It is a cause of great satisfaction that WHO has sponsored this conference. Professor Bettex, Chairman of the Organizing Committee of this conference, Director of the University Children's Hospital in Berne, President of the World Federation of Associations of Paediatric Surgeons, member of the CIOMS Executive Committee: I remember when you started with the idea of this conference and it must be a great satisfaction to you to see it in concrete form. Dr Dogramaci, Executive Director of the International Pediatric Association: your work with the International Pediatric Association is well-known all over the world, and your contribution to WHO as a member of its Executive Board and Advisory Committee for Medical Research must be emphasized. Dr Bankowski, Executive Secretary of the Council for International Organizations of Medical Sciences: I do not have to say how efficient and what a hard worker you are; all in CIOMS are grateful for your constant and permanent dedication to our organization. I am sorry that at the last moment, for very important reasons, Dr Everett Koop, Surgeon General of the United States Public Health Service, found himself unable to attend this meeting. He called and asked us to transmit to all of you his best wishes for a successful conference. He will be very glad to receive the conclusions of the conference, one he considers to have great importance. We had also this morning the message that Dr Robbins could not come, for unexpected resons. As I mentioned before, Dr Gellhorn has very kindly accepted to take his place.

I want to welcome all of you to the XIXth CIOMS Conference, jointly organized with the World Health Organization. Its subject is "Battered Children and Child Abuse". As you know, there has been a real increase in reported cases of child abuse, particularly in industrialized countries, where existing services has permitted the detection of, and response to, cases of child abuse. Many years ago child abuse in the industrial world was thought to be uncommon. Only active public and professional concern has led to the emergence of a truer picture of all forms of child abuse. But it seems that this problem has not remained an isolated North American and European one. Cross-cultural perspectives in the field of child abuse and neglect are largely lacking. Societies are slow to acknowledge and recognize the problem. The definitions vary from culture to culture and evolve

1

over long periods. To command the attention of paediatricians in the United States, Dr Kempe coined the term "the battered child syndrome" at the 1961 annual meeting of the American Academy of Pediatrics. Fortunately, this term has taken hold and has resulted in a significant degree of activity and interest on the part of paediatricians, social agencies, lawyers, police, lay organizations and legislatures. The rights of children and the obligations of the medical profession have been recognized. Very recently the Council of Scientific Affairs of the American Medical Association published some guidelines which had been developed to assist primary care physicians in the identification and management of the various forms of child maltreatment. The International Year of the Child has stimulated world-wide efforts to meet the most urgent needs of children. For the first time in human history the world as a whole has addressed the needs of children wherever they are. I hope that the participants of this conference will gain mutual benefit from their discussions and at the conclusion will offer us a realistic framework for dealing with a tragic international health problem. At this stage, I want to ask Dr Gellhorn to take the chairmanship of this conference. Thank you.

A. Gellhorn, Conference Chairman

Thank you, Dr Belchior. I apologize that Fred Robbins is not here, but I am delighted to have the opportunity to act briefly as his substitute. I would add my comments to Dr Belchior's with regard to congratulating Professor Bettex for having brought us together, for he started in CIOMS six years ago, saying that this was a timely and important topic. It has taken six years to bring us all together — but in what a spot! The Canton of Berne is to be congratulated, and I do not think many of us have been in such beautiful surroundings as this auditorium and the rest of the hospital. I am sure that I speak for all of us in expressing our gratitude. We should like to have a word of support and welcome from Dr Petros-Barvazian of the World Health Organization's Division of Family Health.

B. Roos, Federal Office of Public Health, Berne, Switzerland

Mr. Chairman, very distinguished guests, dear colleagues, ladies and gentlemen. I have the great honour and pleasure to welcome you on behalf of the Swiss Federal authorities to this international conference on Battered Children and Child Abuse and convey their greetings and congratulations. In particular, I congratulate my former colleague, Professor Marcell Bettex, Head of the University Clinic for Paediatric Surgery of the University of Berne, for having so well organized this conference with energy and idealism. We very much appreciate that this very first meeting on this subject, an international meeting on the global level, organized as a joint venture of the Council for International Organizations of Medical Sciences and the World Health Organization, is being held here in Switzerland and especially in our capital, Berne. One of its main goals will be to improve the information about battered children and child abuse — an information gift to all of us, to our authorities, and to the men and women responsible in the different states of this globe, developing and developed countries. We need urgently this information and I am convinced that, first of all, information is perhaps the way we can prevent or, in the future, stop the misery

2

of child abuse. In this whole process of bringing through information to the people, to the families, to the teachers in schools, at university levels, the press, the mass media — television, journalists — have a very important role, because they are the locomotives for the information. I would make only one reservation. When these professionals of the mass media write and talk and demonstrate about these problems of battered children and child abuse, I should like to say to them, "please do it without sensation or making a splash out of an individual case". One can do much harm by tearing out everything of one of these cases, and I think it is the responsibility of these professionals to do it in a very decent and intelligent way. Up to now general practitioners' and paediatricians' efforts have been primarily directed towards improving the physical health of children — that means monitoring the mother and child during pregnancy and delivery, controlling the child's growth and development, improving medical services in schools, including better dentistry, vaccinations, alimentation, sport activities; but perhaps all these activities have not had their whole impact on the problem. We have perhaps forgotten a little bit the social and the cultural-social background of the families. A recent cross-study on the community level in this country conducted by a private organization, the Swiss Association for the Protection of the Child, indicates that the awareness of the problems of battered children and child abuse has in the last few years considerably improved. The study has shown a real amelioration of the structures for prevention and treatment as well as an increased interest of our whole population in broader information. Here I should like to mention the important role that medical societies, professional societies, and private organizations such as the one I mentioned before, play in promoting information. For our small country it is typical that, long before the authorities take steps to change laws and the legal structure, private organizations point the finger to new problems. Also, it is a typical way in Switzerland to go ahead on private initiative and I think that is important.

To end, I would say to you that I hope that during your deliberations and discussions — here in this beautiful lecture-hall — you will reach the goal of all of us for whom the physical, mental and social health of children and adolescents is the most important thing for tomorrow's parents and a priority concern. I welcome you to Berne and wish you all an interesting and rewarding meeting. Thank you.

M. Bettex, Head of Department of Paediatric Surgery, University of Berne, Switzerland

Ladies and Gentlemen, on behalf of the Organizing Committee and also of the Faculty of Medicine of the University of Berne, I welcome you all — speakers, participants, members and guests — to the CIOMS Round Table Conference 1985.

It has been a privilege for the Department of Paediatric Surgery of the Children's Medical Centre in Berne to manage the local arrangements and to work with national and international organizations, and especially with CIOMS and WHO in preparing for the conference.

The Department of Paediatric Surgery is both part of the University of Berne and integrated into the main Bernese hospital, Inselspital. It may sound strange to you but the translation of Inselspital is 'hospital of the isle'. It was founded in

1354 and was once situated on an island in Berne's main river, the Aare. It was formerly a convent.

As host of this conference it is my great pleasure and honour to welcome Dr Petros-Barvazian of WHO's Division of Family Health, who takes the place of Dr Lambo, Deputy Director-General of WHO, who was himself unable to be present today; Dr Belchior, President of CIOMS, from Rio de Janeiro; and Dr Gellhorn, Past-President of CIOMS and now in the State Health Department of the State of New York, who will act here as Chairman of the conference because, as you heard, Dr Robbins was not able to come. I welcome also Dr Beat Roos, Director of the Swiss Federal Office of Public Health in Berne; and Dr Beer, who has not been mentioned until now, of the Beer-Brawand Foundation, who has helped with great generosity in the financing of this conference. Thank you very much, Dr Beer. I thank also all the other sponsors; they are listed in the programme and will also be quoted in the proceedings.

This conference on battered children and child abuse has a long history. In the last 20 years, as you have already heard, we have become more aware of the problem as more and more battered children were referred to the children's hospital and recognized as such by the physicians. All these children were hospitalized in the department of surgery and that is why this conference has been organized by surgeons. The planning began already in 1979, which had been declared the Year of the Child, as already stressed by Dr Belchior. In our unit we encountered many difficulties with this problem — less medical ones than difficulties in dealing with the authorities. This was mainly owing to lack of guidelines for a comprehensive approach. The absence of any guidelines prompted me to propose to CIOMS to convene a conference on this subject. CIOMS is, in my opinion, the best forum for discussing a primarily medical problem with all its social, ethical, moral, administrative, religious, and philosophical implications. CIOMS is also the only organization of a high level where a basic multidisciplinary discussion can be freely held with maximum impact on the governments of the world.

As we began to prepare this conference we soon became aware that the problem of the battered child is only the tip of the iceberg. There are many other forms of child abuse. Child abuse may present itself in quite different ways in industrialized countries and in mainly rural countries. There may be great differences of appreciation of child abuse according to the cultural, philosophical, political and religious backgrounds. Thus we had to enlarge greatly the scope of the conference, as you may have noticed from the programme. However, any discussion about child battering and child abuse should definitely have a goal. This conference should result in the formulation of guidelines on how to handle the problem regionally, nationally and internationally. We profoundly hope that this conference will give the World Health Organization a solid base for elaborating sound policies about this scourge for all the nations of the world.

WELCOME ADDRESS

A. Petros-Barvazian

World Health Organization, Geneva

On behalf of the Director-General of the World Health Organization, Dr Halfdan Mahler, and as Director of the Division of Family Health at World Health Organization Headquarters in Geneva, it gives me much pleasure to welcome all of you to this joint WHO/CIOMS Conference on Battered Children and Child Abuse. Both as a paediatrician and as Director of a programme of which the principal objective is the improvement of the health and well-being of children, I believe that the question of child abuse should have been taken up long ago. For a variety of reasons, not least its inadequate epidemiological definition, it is only now being recognized as the problem that it is.

In taking up this issue, just as in taking up the question of child health in general, we accept responsibility for a major challenge. In all societies children are the most vulnerable members. In some societies and among certain groups they are at an even higher than average risk. Also, although they represent the society of tomorrow and we invest in them our hopes for the future with regard to social and economic development, children in many societies have been sadly neglected and have failed to enjoy the benefits due to them.

Nevertheless, over the past 50 years we have seen improvements. Infant and young child mortality has been effectively controlled in most industrialized regions of the world. In many developing countries, similar progress is already visible and, except in countries particularly affected by the international economic recession, the chances of survival through infancy and childhood have been significantly improved.

The more we look at this problem, however, the more we are concerned with not only achieving better opportunities for survival but also, and of equal importance, assuring a quality of life that enhances the growth and the development of our children. This I see as the second challenge, but one that must be taken up in parallel and as an integral part of our work towards reducing infant and child mortality.

The subject that you have elected to take up in coming to this Conference is fundamental to that challenge. To me, child abuse is not simply or only the problem of child battering or parental neglect. To my thinking, child abuse is anything that deprives the child of the right to healthy growth and development and to the realization of full potential for social development. I do not believe this is too broad a definition, and I should hope that in your deliberations you will place the issue of child beating, child labour, child prostitution, and parental neglect within this broader context of basic human rights and public health.

Even 20 years ago we were still in a position to approach the question of child health from the point of view of specific disease eradication models. Today we face a far more complex global social situation. Demographic patterns have changed dramatically; changes in residential patterns mean that by the end of the century most of the world's population will be urban, and the majority of the urban population will be under the age of 18 years. Perhaps I should not even talk of 'urban', however, because the word has always had connotations of the organized city well served with basic health services. Since the 1960s we have seen a pattern of urban growth emerge that has created a series of slum and squatter settlements and inner-city problem areas which do not do justice to the concept of urban life. It is in these conditions that the stress of trying to survive provokes many of the social problems that eventually result in much of the child abuse and battering that we see in many of our clinics and hospitals. However, in looking at these more immediate problems, which by all means merit all our attention, I would ask you to also address the context in which these problems are emerging and give some thought to how we should all combine our efforts in preparing our public health and social programmes to take up the challenge that is before us.

The World Health Organization looks forward to your recommendations and to your collaboration. The Organization is an extension of your own national programmes and has an obligation to respond to your needs. No issue is more important to it than the achievement of child health, and I would reiterate that child health is more than survival: it is quality of life, the absence of any form of social abuse. The achievement of this goal will call on all our energies, our imagination, and our abilities to look further than the confines of health services *per se* and develop truly multisectoral and multidisciplinary approaches to working with children, families and communities. Please rest assured that the World Health Organization will take up this issue energetically with you.

KEYNOTE ADDRESS

Ihsan Dogramaci

International Pediatric Association

On behalf of the International Pediatric Association I applaud the decision of the World Health Organization and the Council for International Organizations of Medical Sciences to organize a meeting on the important and timely subject of battered children and child abuse.

The problem of child abuse, neglect and mistreatment in general is an old phenomenon and not peculiar to modern society. However, it is the problems of today which we must face and those of tomorrow which we must try to prevent. Our task from an international point of view would seem to me to be to describe the magnitude of the problem and the many forms it takes under different circumstances and among different social groups. We must be grateful to those who have been increasingly active in bringing the problem to our attention and to the attention of public opinion during the past several decades. Among these I should like to pay tribute to Henry Kempe and Henry Silver, who about a quarter of a century ago introduced the term "battered children syndrome" to cover the recurrent fractures and other injuries in infancy and childhood for which parents and baby-sitters or other keepers of those children are directly responsible. The identification of this condition sent a "shock wave" around the world. Kempe and Silver called for paediatricians to be realistic and face the fact that parental criminal neglect and severe physical abuse of children might be more widespread than had ever been imagined and that many of the injuries described in the literature were the result of the mistreatment.

Indeed, some 40 years ago, when I was receiving my paediatric training at the Boston Children's Hospital, Dr Franc Ingraham, neurosurgeon at the same hospital, drew our attention to subdural haematomas, which could be attributed not only to accidental trauma but also to deliberate blows, and he taught us how to recognize the condition clinically. About the same time Dr John Caffey described the presence of multiple fractures of long bones in young children and subdural haematomas in children without bone disease, and he went on to suggest that these conditions might be the result of ill-treatment. It is only 32 years ago that Silverman described what he called "unrecognized skeletal trauma" as identified by X-rays, and suggested that parents who failed to report accidents might indeed have been guilty of causing trauma though quite unaware of having done so, or, if aware of it, simply forgetting it or being reluctant to admit it.

Today there is not much argument among paediatricians, social workers and lawyers about the existence of the battered child syndrome. Our problem now, as I see it, is defining the magnitude of the syndrone, and identifying the factors that contribute to its presentation, predicting high-risk situations, and from there going on to determine how best, and always with the children's interest foremost in our minds, the problem can be dealt with.

Regrettably, data on child abuse are sparse. I understand that only 40 countries regularly compile information on this topic and that among those there are many variations in reporting systems and quality of data. Perhaps it is some indication of how important a problem child abuse is, however, that in 1980 it was conservatively estimated that over 100 babies were battered to death in the United Kingdom by those primarily responsible for them. Another estimated 8,000 children suffered what were called non-accidental injuries. I am sure that, were equivalent data available from other countries, we should see that the problem is not limited to the United Kingdom but rather that it is an extended problem and that it crosses all socioeconomic and cultural demarcations. Indeed, child abuse, including child neglect, exploitation of children and mistreatment of children, crosses all national boundaries. I use the example of the United Kingdom not because the problem is any worse there than elsewhere but rather because the type of attention that has been given to it has promoted the regular reporting of incidents to a greater extent than in other countries. A fairly careful registration by the legal and health care systems there provides us with as good a profile of the problem as we are likely to find today.

No doubt countries and social groups view the problem of child abuse differently. Perhaps they perceive the needs of children differently. In Turkey, for example, in a sample survey carried out between 1980 and 1982 in eight provinces, covering 16,000 children aged 4 to 12 years, Dr Sule Bilir and co-workers found that a large percentage of children had suffered some physical injury as a result of "punishment". The incidence in the 4-6-years age-group was 40.68%; for 7- to 10-year-olds, 33.46%; and for 11- to 12-year-olds, 25.84%. The incidence of injured female children was slightly higher. The incidence was significantly higher in families with more than one child, when the family was an extended one (in contrast to a nuclear family), where the level of education was low and where the parental age was less than 20.

The problem is certainly not a recent one. It has been common to all periods of history. I should hazard a guess that in other times the problem was even more widespread. Certainly, forced labour of young children employed in different types of industries and often for excessively long hours, and the practice of forced marriages and sexual exploitation of children, have been well recorded for many parts of the world and many periods in history. But the incidence of child abuse has been increasing in our modern society. The argument has been put forward that modern-day stress, and the inability of the small family to accommodate to this stress, be it economic, marital, employment-based or whatever, are the main contributing factors, and that child abuse and child beating are simply an expression of parents' inability to deal with the pressures of contemporary urban life. I would not challenge that view; there is, after all, considerable evidence from studies and individual reports to suggest that these types of pressures do indeed contribute to the mistreatment of children. But I would ask why it is, when these pressures are so widespread and do not respect social class or cultural boundaries, that some individuals appear to be far more predisposed to the abuse and exploitation of children than others. The problem, I suspect, is far more complex than simply inability to deal with stress and pressures. It may well have to do with concepts of child-rearing and the experience that the parent had as a child. It may equally have to do with what different cultures expect of children, as regards either economic value or intellectual achievement. It may just as well have to do with whether infants are

8

wanted or not. Inevitably there will be many contributing factors or determinants, which we must certainly address.

We must also seek to describe how best to deal with so-called offenders and how best to help the victim. If, as current data suggest, child abuse is a widespread and almost institutionalized characteristic of our societies, then the task before this conference and other groups who will continue to work in this area is a considerable one. Legal systems, as we all know, move and change slowly. They are often cumbersome and in seeking to help victims impose on them even greater stress. Therefore part of our discussion will necessarily relate to the extent to which child abuse must be viewed as a legal issue or, alternatively, how it can be managed — if at all — by some para-legal mechanism.

Perhaps not all of us see the role of children in the family and society in the same light, or the role of their parents and other people who care for them. This surely is the essence of the problem that we will have to deal with in our discussions. It may well be that our conclusion will be that there is no all-embracing definition of child abuse and neglect, and that the different types of parental and social behaviour *vis-à-vis* children differ so much from one set of social circumstances to another that comparisons are difficult. It may well be that different cultures have different expectations with regard to the whole process of child-rearing and to the authority that the parental system should exert on children. It may well be that under different judicial systems the manner and extent to which child abuse or mistreatment of children can be prosecuted differs so much that different penal systems can ultimately only respond in ways that are culturally relative. But I would argue that there are within this arena a number of universal values, expectations and principles, which can be identified and can help guide our approach to the issue. I would argue that it is not culturally specific to state that children have the right to mental and physical health, to protection from unnecessary trauma, and to the affective type of care that helps ensure psychological well-being. Yet today we realize more and more that parents and others primarily responsible for the upbringing of young children can, and often do, severely neglect or physically harm their own offspring or the children for whom they are responsible. The medical world is growing increasingly aware of the fact that the nature of child neglect and physical abuse is very varied, as is its long-term effect upon the child. We know also that physical harm and neglect are only one side of the coin and that the less visible, less tangible psychological insults which many children experience have a much more lasting and perhaps more devastating effect on the development of the child and on the role the child will go on to play as an adult. Perhaps the organization of systems that incorporate an approach that is fundamentally oriented towards social work and family welfare, with some para-legal character, is called for. This will be a key part of our discussions, since in many countries the whole question remains unexplored to the extent that suggestions and recommendations are required.

From my own point of view, however, it strikes me that we need to know far more about the configurations of familial and societal determinants that can be used in predicting the family that is likely to abuse a child and the child who is destined to become a victim. If we have this type of knowledge in our

9

armamentarium then it should be possible to take preventive action and provide the support that such families need.

Although familial abuse is widely recognized it is still little understood. Those who concern themselves with the practices of child rearing are often surprised to find so much genuine love for the child coupled with frequent and often severe corporal punishment. To the outsider this may seem strangely paradoxical but closer inspection will probably reveal that the intention behind the punishment is the benefit of the child. In such an instance the one inflicting the punishment will be quite unaware that he or she is doing any harm but rather believes that this is a necessary measure if the child is to learn to be obedient, to tell the truth, indeed to be a useful and happy member of society.

Some parents are also quick to punish, encouraged by religious precepts. They take quite literally such sayings as "He that spareth his rod hateth his son; but he that loveth him chasteneth him betimes" (the Bible) and "Beatings are heaven sent" (the Koran).

The mode of punishment is, of course, very much a matter of tradition or experience. The mother who was beaten into obedience as a child is very likely to beat her own child into obedience, just as the mother who was bottle-fed as a baby will very likely bottle-feed her own baby, unless, of course, she is taught otherwise. Just as parents need to be taught the benefits of breastfeeding if this is no longer the tradition, so they need to be taught that there are ways other than corporal punishment of bringing up their children to be well-behaved and respectful, and eventually contented and valuable members of society. No well-meaning parents want to see their children gambling, smoking, stealing or getting involved in practices that will endanger their chances of future happiness, and since their intentions are good it should not be so very difficult to channel their intentions towards something less dangerous and more constructive than corporal punishment.

Let me now turn to the question of child abuse and neglect outside the family, for there are around us a host of broader, more far-reaching examples of child abuse than those occurring in the household. The chronic exposure of young children to war, to involuntary migration, to uprooting, has become so much a part of our 20th century world that perhaps we have ceased to see it as the insidious problem it is with regard to both the physical and the emotional development of children.

There are two areas in child abuse that I should now like to dwell upon. One is child labour. The International Labour Office estimates that in the world as a whole 52 million children aged less than 15 are working; however, we should remember that, since statistics cover only those youngsters who have a fixed and permanent job, those who work only occasionally are generally excluded, with the result that the figure is higher than the one estimated.

We do not have to look far for the reason why these young people work. It is poverty that pressures families into trying to increase their resources through the assistance, meagre though this may be, which even very young children can provide. Equally, many children must provide directly for their own needs. Employers are quick to cash in on the advantages of the cheap labour thus afforded by economic necessity, and governments of developing countries are forced to condone a practice which, for the sake of economy, they may not condemn. There is, however, much in the working conditions and practice of child and adolescent employment which should be condemned. In most cases, children and young adolescents work in conditions which were designed not for them but for adults. Frequently, they are employed in unsanitary premises, in contact with toxic substances, or, if out of doors, without suitable protection from the weather. Their work is all too often too strenuous and puts too much strain on still developing bodies. The child that works should at least be given a shorter working day and allowed more holidays, but all too often the reverse is the case. Many children are forced to work a 10-hour day and a six- or even a seven-day week. Often there is virtually no pay or it is at best absurdly inadequate. There is neither decent accommodation nor adequate nourishment to balance out to some extent the effort required in the working day, with the result that the child's health is almost certainly irrevocably undermined.

Not only are long working hours detrimental to the child's physical health; also they have a negative, often destructive effect on the well-being and development of the personality, particularly if the child is working away from the family. The child is then deprived of a harmonious family life, has insufficient time for play and cultural activities and is frequently exposed to social risks of one kind or another.

The other important area I wish to bring to your attention is that of sexual abuse and juvenile prostitution. Sexual abuse of children is perpetrated frequently by members of the victim's family and acquaintances of the child, and much less frequently by strangers. In a sample of 930 women in San Francisco 16% reported at least one experience of intra-familial abuse before the age of 18 years and 12% reported at least one such incident before the age of 14. Extra-familial abuses were even more frequent, having occurred to 31% of the women before the age of 18 and to 20% before they had turned 14. Of all these abuses, only 2% of those within the family and 6% of extra-familial cases had ever been reported to the police. Fathers and uncles are the most usual perpetrators, but brothers, first cousins and even grandfathers also are implicated. Female perpetrators of sexual abuse of girls are also not unheard of.

Let me turn now to the problems of juvenile prostitution, the predisposing factors of which are many and various. Young people who have not enjoyed the security of a happy family background, and who have been neglected and rejected, naturally yearn for attention and approval and, never having known genuine love, may feel that prostitution or sexual relations can give them what they need. Further, if, as is often the case, their school-work has not been good, and they have developed no skills and consequently have apparently no other way of making a living, these young people too easily believe that they have no alternative. The initiative may come from the youngster, but equally it may come from an organized ring.

In the larger cities in particular, there are many organized prostitution rings holding out the promise of support, security and affection to youngsters who, for various reasons, have left their homes. Food and a roof over their heads are enough to tempt a youngster at a loose end. Many of these boys and girls may be no strangers to sexual exploitation, having suffered sexual abuse or incest before leaving home. They may already have learned that prostitution can provide the material necessities of life and are easily caught up in the web of a "protector" who exploits their need for attention and material support. It is often extremely difficult to pry the victims away from these surroundings in the face of both the

11

professional criminal environment in which they find themselves and their own resistance to rehabilitation. Besides, such surroundings are breeding grounds for alcoholism and drug abuse, which make escape even more difficult.

After so much emphasis on child abuse, it is also worth remembering that sometimes a diagnosis of child abuse may be unfounded. In the case of a young infant it is obviously very difficult, perhaps even impossible, to determine whether certain injuries are the result of a fall or of abuse. Further, how are we to distinguish between terms like carelessness and gross carelessness, neglect and wilful or criminal neglect? Some people, faced with what could be a case of child abuse, tend to be governed by their emotions and jump to the conclusion that it is indeed a case of child abuse without first considering whether there are not other possible explanations.

This is particularly true when the child in question is dead. We should never forget that the death or serious illness of a child is a truly traumatic experience, and that the questioning of anyone close to the child might well produce an unpleasant reaction. If, coupled with the shock of the child's death, a parent comes up against an unjust accusation of child abuse, it is little wonder if he or she behaves in a manner that is far from calm and controlled. Even medical staff, who should be trained to cope with such a situation and, moreover, have less at stake, find it hard enough to remain civilized when unjustly blamed for neglect of a patient. This is a matter that must be faced in a positive and constructive manner. One measure that I should like to suggest is that there should always be expert, trained consultants at hand so that, should it be necessary to question those close to or responsible for the child, this can be done in as calm and objective a manner as possible so as to give the least possible occasion for offence.

In addition to the emotional grounds for making a wrong diagnosis of child abuse, we should also remember the clinical grounds. I refer to the normal post-mortem changes that set in after death, but with which many physicians are unfamiliar. There is for example the blood-streaked fluid which may issue from nose or mouth; this is, of course, a combination of fluid from the lungs and the blood of ruptured nasal capillaries, but the inexperienced physician can easily mistake it for the result of a facial trauma, in other words as evidence of child abuse. Sometimes the natural settling of the blood in dependent parts of the body has been misconstrued as bruising; such discolouring will disappear during the early hours after death if lightly pressed, but later it is hard, even impossible, to distinguish it from bruising. A third change that may lead to misunderstanding is the distortion of the normal anatomical features, the result of the subcutaneous fat of the body congealing as the body temperature falls.

These are some reflections that I want to share with you as we begin our deliberations at this exceedingly important conference. May I reiterate my appreciation to both WHO and CIOMS for convening this meeting and also for giving me the opportunity to be with you.

NATURE AND MAGNITUDE
OF THE PROBLEM

CHILD MALTREATMENT AND ITS PRESENTATION IN INDUSTRIALIZED COUNTRIES

Richard Krugman*

My perspective of child abuse and neglect is derived from a clinical base, since I am a pediatrician and work every day with children and families. The C. Henry Kempe National Center for the Prevention and Treatment of Child Abuse and Neglect is a multidisciplinary center of 29 professionals. Last year our child protection team cared for over 400 children at University Hospital, over 150 families at our Child Diagnostic Treatment Center, and many other families in a "Third Party" sexual abuse (by strangers) programme. We also have a therapeutic pre-school programme for sexually abused three- and four-year olds.

Dr Dogramaci has covered some of the history of this field and I would encourage you to read a paper by Dr Margaret Lynch of Great Britain, entitled *Child Abuse before Kempe*, in Volume 9, No. 1 of Child Abuse and Neglect, the International Journal. She points out that abuse and neglect have been occurring for centuries. Dr Dogramaci referred to the Biblical phrase "Spare the rod, spoil the child". I would remind you that these are the words of Solomon, who, if you look at the outcome of his sons, was probably somewhat abusive to them. His son, Rheoboam, was a most vicious individual who wreaked havoc and killed many women and children. The Bible nowhere attributes to God other than a nurturing attitude to children, and perhaps, rather than listen to some of the kings who were quoted, we ought to take that lesson. In Roman Law there is the concept of the *patria potestia*, which meant that children were property and fathers ruled. Whatever father said was so. Soranus, a Greek physician in 300 A.D., wrote a textbook called *Gynecology* which had a section that described which children should be kept and which should be disposed of. Among the children that Soranus felt should be kept were children who were perfect and of good temper. Those who were of poor temper, or had congenital deformities should be disposed of. In describing how to choose a wet-nurse, he also gave what may have been the first description of what John Caffey, the radiologist, later described as the infant whip-lash shaking syndrome. He said that a wet-nurse should be a woman of even temper, because if she were of poor temper she would shake and tremble and let the baby fall from her hands when it cried. The baby would fall on its head, get water on the brain and grow up to be a retarded child. This type of response (as you will see when I describe later how we analyse physical abuse today) to a child's crying has been noted throughout centuries to lead to abusive assaults on a child. Lynch also describes the work of a Geneva pediatrician, Theofis Bonnet, who also described angry wet-nurses and their effect on children.

It is always easier to accept that some one from outside the family will be the one who will abuse a child, rather than someone inside. Probably the first physician to notice it within the family was Ambroise Tardieu, a French physician who in 1860 described 32 cases that were clearly battered children.

* Director, C. Henry Kempe National Center for the Prevention and Treatment of Child Abuse and Neglect, 1205 Oneida Street, Denver, Colorado 80220, U.S.A.

There were 18 deaths. Many of the children were burned or suffocated. He described the frozen watchfulness of the children, who were hypervigilant because they were never sure when they were going to be abused. However, his paper was ignored and then, as Dr. Dogramaci pointed out, John Caffey in 1946 described the association of multiple fractures with subdural haematoma. Fred Silverman in 1953 said those fractures were trauma, that we should stop looking for congenital defects and defects of calcium metabolism or other problems as the cause. In 1955 Drs Evans and Wooley said that children with these fractures had suffered inflicted injury. Again, however, these papers were ignored and it was not until 1961 when Henry Kempe presented his paper, *The Battered Child Syndrome*, that people listened.

My purpose today then will be to define various forms of the problem. Dr Obikeze has defined the many aspects of abuse. I will try to build on that, but in addition to my clinical perspective I will also attempt to look at abuse and neglect from the child's viewpoint. We ought not spend time trying to define what abuse and neglect is. In my opinion, abuse and neglect is defined community by community, state by state, country by country, culture by culture, and society by society around the world. What is considered abuse in Denver, Colorado may or may not be considered abuse in another part of the United States, and may or may not be considered abuse elsewhere. What *is* important is that individuals among the public and professionals will define child abuse from a child's perspective in their own culture. These individuals should try to see whether a child is being harmed by *whatever* we are talking about, whether it is physical abuse, sexual abuse, emotional abuse or emotional neglect.

Dr Kempe in his original paper estimated that there might be as many as 447 cases of battered child syndrome in the United States then. That today represents an eight-hour total, for the figure in 1983 was 1,007,658 reported cases, in 1984, about 400,000, and in 1985, about 1,700,000. The estimates vary, for our data systems are not very good. The perpetrator of the abuse is a parent in 92% of cases, and the most prevalent type of abuse is deprivation and neglect (about 58%). About 25–40% in 1983 was physical abuse and about 2% sexual abuse, but sexual abuse was up to 7% in the 1984 data and 13% in 1985, and it is very underreported. In Colorado, 27% of all cases of reported abuse and neglect are sexual abuse; it is therefore an increasingly recognized problem.

Of reported families, 40% are headed by a single person, and in 40% the head is unemployed. Children at risk include those who are unsupervised. In the United States more than 2 million are left alone in the home while parents work. The reports of child abuse increase with lack of supervision. Johnson County, Kansas is one example, where as children are left unsupervised more tend to be reported for abuse and neglect. Clearly, other children who are at risk are those who are born to parents afflicted with alcoholism, of whom there are 28 million, perhaps the most identifiable cause of child maltreatment. Children in foster-care are another high-risk group. We have over 500,000 children who need secure homes. Half a million children in foster-care in the United States, the great majority, are there because of abuse and neglect, not because they have been orphaned. Other children at risk are those who are subject to corporal punishment. A study by the Department of Education revealed that corporal punishment was administered over a million times in 77,000 schools, from kindergarten through twelfth grade. Another at-risk group, particularly as

15

regards sexual abuse as well as physical abuse, are the children of divorced parents: 40% of children in the United States will try to cope with the divorce of parents, 70% will have that experience twice, and many of these children who then find themselves with boy-friends or girl-friends of the parent with whom they are living are at increased risk, being in a non-biological home, of physical or sexual abuse.

When we look at physical abuse clinically, the question is— are we dealing with accidental or non-accidental injury? There is evidence in the work of various investigators, including the Newbergers in Boston and others, of a clear overlap and a clear link between neglect and accidental injury in children. And yet, when we are faced with a clinical case of injury, we have to decide whether it was accidental or not. The best way of coming to this decision is to take a detailed history of the parents, and of course this has to be done in emergency rooms. The key feature in differentiation is the discrepant history. The history given by the parent or other guardian does not fit with what we see in the child. For example, a parent will say that the child fell off the couch, and the child has a skull fracture on both sides of the head. Clearly, the child cannot get bilateral skull fractures from falling off the couch. The second feature is delay in seeking care. Very often when parents see children have accidental injury in our industrialized societies they tend to rush for care where care is available. If there is a health system and a child does have an injury, most parents feel protective and rush to have their child treated.

Abusive families seem to be in crisis always, and often a crisis precipitates the abusive event, and the child always seems to have a behaviour that triggers the assault. The most common trigger in infants under one year of age is inconsolable crying, children who cry and cry and cry, and they are finally beaten or shaken. Over one year of age the most common trigger we see clinically is loss of bowel or bladder control: children wet the bed or soil their pants, and they are beaten or burned for it. In all of the families who have been seen at our Center over 27 years, when an adequate history is taken we find that the abusers have a prior history of inadequate nurture as children and most often they were abused in the same way as they abuse their children. That repetition of the cycle is of great importance in planning treatment and prevention programmes. Of course, not all abused children grow up to be abusive adults. No one has yet done the kinds of prospective longitudinal studies that are needed to discover how many abused children are at risk of repeating that cycle — we hope such data will become available. We also see parents with unrealistic expectations, social isolation in the families, a pattern of increased severity of injury in children who are abused: they come to us first with a bruise, then with a fracture, then with multiple fractures, then with enormous subdural hematomas and death. They may go to many hospitals and many care agencies as well, because they don't want anyone to notice that pattern. The physical features of abuse have been well described, but whether it is bruises or burns, head injuries, abdominal injuries, or fractures, there are certain medical features that are, if not diagnostic, certainly suggestive of abuse. Certain patterns of bruises or injuries rarely occur accidentally — a pinch-mark on the end of the penis, a bruise in the shape of electric cords or belts, burns, head injuries, abdominal injuries including duodenal hematomas and pancreatic injuries, and various types of fractures such as metaphyseal chip fractures or spiral fractures in infancy. Associated social features in these families include poverty, adolescent parents, prematurity, and a pattern of family violence and unemployment. Each of these is a feature that increases stress in families but does not itself cause abuse and neglect. Poverty, for example, can cause financial stress and can lead to problems in families. An unemployed parent is around the home more than an employed one. But the reality is that there are many unemployed families and many parents of premature babies, and many adolescent parents, and many very poor parents, who take wonderful care of their children. Poverty alone, or unemployment alone, does not explain abuse, but as an associated sociological factor it makes it more likely that some one who is predisposed to abusing a child, because of his or her own childhood experience, will repeat that cycle.

With regard to sexual abuse there has been a dramatic increase in recognition. We are now in a period of increasing understanding of sexual abuse, in part because we understood physical abuse first. In the late 1960s in our country many women said "wait a minute, it's not just children who are battered, women are battered too". As individuals began to work with battered women they began to hear from many of them that they had been sexually abused as children. This led many pediatricians to wonder why, if these women were sexually abused as children when they saw them in their offices and clinics ten years ago, they did not know that. The answer is that they did not know because they did not ask. They did not ask because they did not know to ask. In sexual abuse, unlike most other problems that come into a medical office, unless one asks, one will not get the answer; children are coerced into keeping a secret and they will never tell what has been going on because they are helpless and afraid. So, for decades we never asked and we never saw cases. Now that public awareness is greater, we are asking more. Also there are television programes and books and programmes in schools, that are asking all the time, and the answer from children is that it is happening. The number of cases seen has gone up dramatically over the last decade — a 576% increase in national reported statistics over a 10-year period. It is this increase that is flooding our system and giving us a lot to deal with.

The presentation of sexual abuse in childhood is variable. One is that children give an early warning. They make generalized statements. They will walk up to their neighbors and say "there is a lot of raping and molesting going on in California", and they are living in Colorado. This is a way of trying to open the conversation. If the neighbor says "don't talk about such things", they won't. They will shut down again. But if the neighbor says, "tell me, has that happened to you?" — the child may so 'no' at first but then later will tell because he or she has not been chastized. Another form of early warning may be in behaviour, where a three-or four-year-old may act out sexually with dolls or other children of their age. Still another may take the form of direct statements. They may also have medical illnesses. We are now recognizing a large number of medical illnesses that may be indicators of sexual abuse in children — recurrent urinary tract infections, enuresis and encopresis (loss of bladder or bowel control), or sexually transmitted diseases. When we see these medical illnesses, it has to alert us to ask the children what is going on.

We see also behavioural changes in children as a form of presentation: school problems, nightmares, night terrors, sexual acting-out, running away, suicidal behaviour, promiscuity, and pregnancy. A very important area to be aware of is children having sexual activity with younger children — 20% of the sexual abuse

17

reported in the United States is perpetrated by adolescents, many of whom have been sexually abused themselves and are turning on younger children as the first manifestation of their sexual abuse. Finally, many problems do not appear until later — in mental health clinics and psychiatrists' offices with adults who have problems with sexual relationships, marital problems, divorces, depression, drug- and alcohol-related problems, and others. The presentations are quite varied, therefore. The key feature is if we see these types of symptoms, while they are not all specific for sexual abuse, that we must give the opportunity to the child or the adult to disclose what happened. They cannot, for a variety of reasons that have been well described in the literature, come right out and say, "that happened to me". It is rare for a child to come walking into an office and say, "I have been sexually abused, help me" or for a parent to come in and say the same.

There are specific medical findings in sexual abuse, Dr Hendrika Cantwell in Denver has found and published in *Child Abuse and Neglect, The International Journal* (Vol. 7:2) a paper where she noted that, on vaginal inspection of pre-pubertal girls, an enlarged vaginal introitus greater than 4 mm was associated with sexual abuse 80% of the time. She has another paper coming out in 1986 which extends and corroborates her earlier findings. There are some who are doing magnifying colposcopy to examine the external genitalia of children, and they are finding some features that are suggestive as well, but these studies have not yet been well enough controlled for us to say with certainty that everyone should be using colposcopy. There are laboratory findings which indicate that children who have venereal disease — gonorrhoea or syphilis — are sexually abused until proven otherwise. If one finds with forensic studies the presence of sperm or alkaline phosphatase, as is done in rape examinations, this too is diagnostic.

Dr David Finkelhor of New Hampshire in his recent book *Child Sexual Abuse Theory and Practice* describes a "four pre-conditions model" for how sexual abuse occurs. He includes both individual traits and social and cultural traits. The first pre-condition is that an individual has to have the motivation to sexually abuse. The second is to overcome certain internal inhibitions. The third is to overcome external inhibitors; the most common external inhibitor to sexual abuse in a family is the presence of a protective spouse; if that spouse is gone, or not able to protect, abuse occurs. The fourth pre-condition is resistance of children. If all four are overcome sexual abuse is likely to occur. Unfortunately, many of the efforts to prevent sexual abuse concentrate on the fourth pre-condition; they are designed to try to keep children from being sexually abused.

With regard to emotional abuse, the best work has been done by Dr James Garbarino, now of the Erickson Institute in Chicago. Emotional abuse is defined as the chronic rejecting, ignoring, criticizing and intimidating or terrorizing of a child. It erodes the child's self-esteem and it leads to a wide variety of symptoms in children. Most are non-specific anxiety symptoms, such as nightmares, night terrors, enuresis, encopresis and many of the things we see in the presentation of sexual abuse as well. Emotional abuse is very difficult to understand, for there are no bruises and no scars. Where we have looked to county and state governments to provide protective services they are so swamped with physical and sexual abuse that they cannot deal with emotional abuse.

Emotional neglect in infants is manifested as non-organic failure to thrive, which we define as a syndrome characterized first by a disordered infant-caregiver interaction and secondly by growth failure due to inadequate energy intake, in the absence of organic disease. Studies on children with non-organic failure to thrive prove this to be one of the most difficult areas for professionals to deal with. Published data show a clear relation between physical abuse and non-organic failure to thrive. Elmer and Gregg in 1967 found that, of children who were diagnosed as physically abused, 55% also had non-organic failure to thrive and on later follow-up 25% still did. In other studies, 16 to 55% of children who are seen for physical abuse have non-organic failure to thrive. Further, the sequels of non-organic failure to thrive are quite significant. Most children followed for three to five years still are below the third percentile for weight, height and head circumference; half have behaviour problems; half have developmental retardation; 10% have psychiatric disturbance; 33% have school difficulties. The mortality of non-organic failure to thrive is significant and I think very unappreciated. The study by Oates and Hufton in 1977 was a six-year follow-up of 24 children. Two were dead. In another one- to three-year follow-up study, five of 22 children were lost to follow-up but of the remaining 17 two were dead. No details were given. In Clare Haynes' study at our Center, a one-to three-year follow-up of 50 hospitalized children, two had died in three years. These are children who disappear from the system and most are physically abused and most come from about 10% of mothers. Specifically, in Haynes' study of children who failed to thrive, 44 were available for follow-up three years later: two were dead, five had been physically abused or neglected, 29 still had retarded growth, 26 had delayed development and 10 were not in their biologic home. Emotional neglect is a significant problem and one which we have not come to grips with. Another interesting feature of her study was that 40% of the mothers of children who had been hospitalized with non-organic failure to thrive disclosed to the interviewer for the first time that they had been victims of incest. We see then, that physical abuse, sexual abuse and emotional neglect are interrelated and are not easily separable. In fact, emotional unavailability is probably the common thread for what is seen in physical sexual abuse.

Briefly then, I think we need to address this issue in stages. When Henry Kempe coined the phrase "battered children syndrome" the main purpose was to stimulate professional and public awareness. He was successful. The same thing is now true in our country of sexual abuse. Over the past seven years we have had a dramatic increase in public awareness. In other countries the increase has been somewhat slower. We need descriptions of the medical, social, legal, and mental health aspects of recognition. We need to stimulate treatment programmes as an offshoot of that descriptive activity, and finally, in the growth and development of a society's approach to abuse programmes, the emergence of prevention programmes. I would estimate that we know about 90% of what we need to know in the area of physical abuse with regard to recognition, treatment and prevention. What we don't have yet is the application of that knowledge in nation-wide or world-wide programmes. In sexual abuse we probably know 90% of what we need to know to be able to recognize the problem, although we do not yet have the dissemination of that knowledge throughout the world. We know about half of what we need to know, or less, for treatment. I regret that we do not have more data about the treatment of families who are involved in sexual abuse because there is a great debate and a great uncertainty as to whether sexually abusive parents should go to jail or get mental health treatment. We know relatively little about prevention, although that has not stopped us from developing 177 different prevention programmes in the U.S. In emotional abuse and neglect we know very little and have an enormous amount to do.

In conclusion, let me make some observations. Much has been learned medically, socially and legally over the last 25 years since Dr Kempe's paper, but much more remains to be done. We have a paucity of prospective data, which makes it very difficult for us to know what we are really doing.

Secondly, as I said before, I think the last thing we need to do is to define abuse. Our Government spent millions of dollars trying to define abuse and neglect, and was unable to do it. I would hope that the rest of the world does not try to follow suit. Because of vast differences in our cultures, in our countries and in our societies, approaches to child abuse very often become a political problem. You should not look to our approaches in the United States and automatically copy them. But neither should you ignore our experience. I think what we have learned is that in our country there are many social and cultural aspects to the problem, including family violence, advertisements which seem to have been designed by pedophiliacs, television, the presence of guns and firearms, and a glorification of violence, which may not be present in your own society. However, that does not mean you do not have battered children, and it does not mean that you do not have sexually abused children. If you begin to look, you will begin to find it. We have made some progress. At the 7th National Conference on Child Abuse, in Chicago, Drs Gelles and Strauss presented data indicating that family violence had decreased in severity in the United States over the last five years. Those of us working in pediatrics were already aware of that. The battered child that Henry Kempe described in 1961 is a child now rarely seen in the United States. We see many cases of physical abuse, but mostly children with burns and bruises. We rarely see the children with multiple fractures, subdural hematomas and burns whom Henry saw 25 years ago, and I believe the reason that we do not see those children is that we have a dramatic increase in public and professional awareness, intervention, reporting and getting those children into a safe place and providing services to the family so that the child does not get rebattered. That is progress in spite of an increase from 447 to 1,007,000 cases.

Finally we must all maintain perspective. In many ways deciding to work in this area is like trying to empty the ocean with a bucket — you take a bucket at a time and you pour it behind you, and years later when you look at the ocean the waves are still crashing in. If you keep looking at the ocean, you will think that nothing has happened but, if you look behind you, you see a nice pool of water. Each of those buckets represents one child or one family who has been helped and that makes this work worthwhile.

Now I will close with a story that Ray Helfer tells about working with Henry Kempe. It is worth remembering when one is working in this area. Ray was absolutely inundated with work one day and, as Henry Kempe tended to do, he handed him a piece of paper and on it was written "take care of this". Henry had been asked by the University of Chicago Press to develop a book entitled *The Battered Child*, which was to come out in 1968. Henry wrote on the letter from the University of Chicago Press, "Ray, take care of this" and he sent it to Ray. Well, Ray came storming up to Henry's office and he said, "Henry, I've got medical students in the clinic I'm supposed to teach because you put me in charge of the third-year students, I've got battered kids on the ward I'm supposed to see, I've got two subpoenas to go to court in the next two days, I've got a research paper due for publication, I'm supposed to prepare my abstract for the American Pediatric Society, and now you tell me to take care of this. How do you expect me to do all of those things?" And without looking up Henry said, "one at a time". That is precisely how we need to approach this particular problem. Whether it is child by child, family by family, profession by profession, or country by country, if we take them one at a time, perhaps 10 or 15 years from now we will be able to look back and have much more information.

CHILD MALTREATMENT IN NON-INDUSTRIALIZED COUNTRIES: A FRAMEWORK FOR ANALYSIS

D. S. Obikeze*

Edwin Reubens (1967) has listed five reasons for societies to devote special attention to children and young persons:

a) the special needs of children and youth;
b) the special interrelationships among these needs;
c) the unique relationship of the new generation to the evolving society;
d) the special dependency and vulnerability of children;
e) the special organizational problems of juvenile care. (Reubens 1967:4)

The fourth item on this list, namely, the special dependency and vulnerability of children, is, to my mind, the most crucial for this conference. It provides the rationale, the raison d'être, for this gathering.

Of all the disadvantaged "minority" groups in human society — the women, the aged, the handicapped, refugees, etc. — children appear to be the weakest and most helpless. That this is so is not difficult to see: the reason is both biological and social. In general, while childhood lasts, children do not participate in, or directly influence, decision-making, even in matters of vital interest to them. At the same time, society demands of them absolute obedience and total submission to the authority and dictates of their adult guardians and parents. It is this situation of voiceless minority that makes children particularly vulnerable to attack and abuse by the other groups in a society (Cantwell, 1979).

However, recognizing that the continued existence of society depends on the survival of the younger generation, all human societies have taken steps to protect their children from undue exploitation and abuse by setting the limits of acceptable levels of conduct to children. In the developing countries, this almost instinctive concern for the welfare of the young finds expression in the folklore, beliefs, mores, traditions and customary practices of the different peoples. In the industrialized countries, it is exhibited in various legal provisions, legislation and statutes, and in the creation of specialized agencies and professional organizations devoted to ensuring the protection and welfare of children.

Thus while the concept of child abuse or maltreatment appears to be common to all human groups, what acts are regarded as abusive are culturally determined. They differ considerably over time and space, and in form and range of manifestations, according to societal norms and value orientations. As Cantwell has put it, "apart from physical violence, there are other manifestations of maltreatment such as abandonment and exploitation, both within and outside the family, which, according to the country concerned, may require more immediate response and priority" (1979: 133).

This paper focuses on child maltreatment and abuse in non-industrialized countries. More specifically, it examines how this phenomenon is perceived and

---

* Department of Sociology/Anthropology, University of Nigeria, Nsukka, Anambra State, Nigeria

defined in these societies; the sociocultural, economic and political forces and conditions that engender it; its various dimensions and ramifications; and possible measures to improve security and the quality of life for children.

Concept clarification/definition

Any attempt to define and operationalize the concept of child abuse in the context of the non-industrialized nations runs into serious problems because, as Kempe and Helfer have observed, "our understanding of this perplexing social problem is limited in that it is based almost entirely on studies in Western nations . . . " (1980:21). Put differently, almost all the available literature on this subject is based on the Western industrialized nations partly because in most of the non-industrialized countries child abuse of the type that happened in North America and Europe in the late 1950s and early 1960s has not yet been "discovered". Although child abuse occurs in the non-industrialized countries, it has not yet been recognized as a significant social malady requiring national and international joint action.

Related to this problem is an even more generalized one, namely lack of clarity and specificity in the use of terms and concepts. As Sweet and Resick have pointed out, "there is a certain confusion in literature on maltreatment of children because of a lack of clearly defined terms" (1979:40). All too often, one finds such terms as "child battering", "child neglect", "child abuse", "child maltreatment", "physical abuse" being used by different authors to refer to the same or very similar occurrences (v. Cantwell, 1979; Sweet and Resick, 1979; Kempe and Helfer, 1980; Braden, 1981).

Perhaps, one fundamental cause of this lack of unanimity in the use of terms is the multidisciplinary nature of the subject, with the result that authors based in a particular discipline refer to certain "pet" terms which they consider reflect their perspective. Thus, for instance, medical writers may prefer the word "battering" since it focuses on the child's poor physical state. To the social worker, the term "child neglect" may be more attractive, since it implies a need of social work. Similarly, a psychologist or psychiatrist, with an eye on the child's emotional state, may prefer to use the term "child abuse". This confusion does not conduce to growth of knowledge in the field since it is "difficult to interpret and compare findings across studies investigating incidence of maltreatment, suspected causes, characteristics of perpetrators and victims . . . when vague and contradictory criteria are used in attaching labels such as 'abuse' and 'neglect' to particular cases" (Sweet and Resick, 1979:40).

Therefore, the first task in analysing and discussing the phenomenon of child maltreatment in non-industrialized nations is to attempt a standardization and operational definition of key concepts. In doing so, I have created no new concepts, but rather synthesized and more precisely redefined existing terms.

Child maltreatment. This is a generic, all-embracing, term which covers not only parental acts but also actions (as well as omissions) of other individuals, groups, organizations, or institutions, or of society at large, which "jeopardise the physical, social, mental, or moral development of the child to some degree" (Veillard-Cybulska, 1975:29). Put another way, it covers all behaviour patterns, whether or not sanctioned by law and custom, which are in some way injurious to the child's health or social, economic, emotional or moral well-being.

Child abuse. Adopting the views of Giovannoni (1971), child abuse is defined as parental acts that constitute a misuse (i.e. abuse) or exploitation of the rights of parents and other guardians to control and discipline children under their care. It occurs when a parent or guardian knowingly misuses a privileged position over the child to commit acts "of non-economic nature" which are not in tune with the societal norms and which are detrimental to the child's health and well-being. Child abuse takes a variety of forms:

(a) Physical abuse (physical violence or non-accidental injury): According to D. G. Gil (1970), "Physical abuse of children is the intentional, non-accidental use of physical force . . . on the part or of a parent or other caretaker interacting with a child in his care, aimed at hurting, injuring or destroying the child".

(b) Social abuse: This results from acts that are detrimental to the child's proper development as a full and functioning member of society. These include all forms of discrimination and denials of rights and privileges on the basis of age, sex, illegitimacy, race, ethnicity or family status.

(c) Emotional (psychological) abuse: This results from acts that militate against the child's adequate personality development. These may involve "continual scape-goating, terrorizing and rejection" (Schmitt, 1980:869).

(d) Sexual abuse: According to Schmitt (1980), this may be defined as any sexual misuse of the child by a care-taking or family related adult. Sexual abuse includes incest, oral-genital contact, sodomy, molestation, digital manipulation, etc.

(e) Drug abuse: "This is deliberate drugging of children by adult caretakers" with sedatives intended for use by adults or by sharing narcotics and alcoholic drinks with them (Schmitt 1980:869).

Child neglect. Child neglect, or "passive child abuse" as Braden (1981) calls it, occurs when parents or guardians fail to perform duties and obligations, "including those of supervision, nurturance, and protection" which fall within limits of their ability and social circumstances (Sweet and Resick 1979:41). It includes denial of food, shelter, clothing, medical care, education and toilet facilities or total abandonment.

Child battering. Child battering differs from physical abuse only in degree or severity. As Schmitt (1980) suggests, any physical abuse (or non-accidental injury) that requires medical attention and treatment or leaves bruises is child battering.

Child exploitation. Child exploitation is a form of child abuse which yields some economic benefits to the perpetrator or someone else. More specifically, child exploitation occurs when a child is made to engage in some gainful productive activity or service which is detrimental to its physical, social, psychological and moral development. It includes, among other acts, child labour and child prostitution.

Physical punishment as a disciplinary measure (harsh punishment)

A fine distinction has to be made between punishment, as a disciplinary

24

measure, and maltreatment. Appropriate punishment for bad behaviour as a means of disciplining children is a virtuous child-rearing practice valued and cultivated in all cultures. However, punishment as a disciplinary measure, whether physical or non-physical, becomes maltreatment when:

(a) it is too harsh or severe for the child's age, or physical and emotional state;
(b) it runs counter to the community's norms and value orientations, and
(c) it is in any way detrimental to the child's well-being and proper development.

The Analytical Framework

In this and subsequent sections an attempt will be made to apply the key concepts defined above to the analysis and description of child maltreatment in non-industrialized countries. On account of the extreme complexity of this problem, I have prepared an analytical framework (Fig. 1) to facilitate a systematic and comprehensive treatment of the subject.

Operational levels

I find it helpful "to distinguish between levels at which the cultural and social (also environmental) context come into play in defining" and analysing maltreatment (Kempe and Helfer, 1980). In non-industrialized societies there are three such levels:

Level I, which may be called the global level. Maltreatment is traceable to structural conditions in the world socioeconomic order. Children in the non-industrialized countries are victims of structural defects in the world system. Amelioration or eradication of maltreatment can be achieved only by a radical transformation of society or a restructuring of the world order.

At Level II, the cultural level, maltreatment refers to "child-rearing practices that may be viewed as acceptable by one group but as unacceptable or even abusive and neglectful by another" (Kempe and Helfer, 1980:22). Child maltreatment is institutionalized and the child is a victim of harsh disciplinary or other customary practices approved by societal norms but, nonetheless, detrimental for the child. Efforts at dealing with the problem will be best directed towards changing societal norms and child-rearing values.

At Level III, the individual level, maltreatment is "idiosyncratic departure from culturally and socially acceptable standards" (Kempe and Helfer, 1980:22). Efforts to eradicate it at this level must be directed at the parents or guardians.

"Global" child maltreatment

At the global level, child maltreatment in non-industrialized societies may be grouped into two categories, "societal" and "non-societal". Societal maltreatment is generated by conditions in the social structure. Prominent among these are underdevelopment, poverty, ignorance and deprivation, which most of these countries share. With underdevelopment and poverty goes scarcity of vital resources. Whenever there is scarcity, children as a voiceless minority group are among the first to suffer maltreatment — denials and deprivations. This is

25

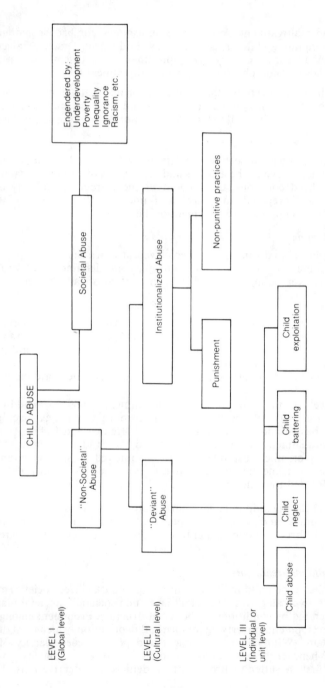

Figure 1: Child abuse: analytical model.

LEVEL I
(Global level)

LEVEL II
(Cultural level)

LEVEL III
(Individual or
unit level)

CHILD ABUSE

Societal Abuse

"Non-Societal"
Abuse

Engendered by:
Underdevelopment
Poverty
Inequality
Ignorance
Racism, etc.

Institutionalized Abuse

"Deviant"
Abuse

Non-punitive practices

Punishment

Child
exploitation

Child
battering

Child
neglect

Child abuse

clearly demonstrated in the level of hunger, malnutrition and premature deaths among children in Third World countries. As Lester Brown (1975) has rightly observed, "in many poor countries of Asia, Africa and Latin America, children under six years of age account for half of all deaths that occur" (1975:6). In a recent study in the Philippines, "nutritionists found that over 80% of all children under the age of six were underweight" (Brown 1975:4). By 1970 in Senegal, 272 of every 1,000 babies died before their fifth birthday. For Cameroon, the figure was 194 (Hobcraft 1985:4). In India and Pakistan 130 of every 1,000 live-born children die before their first birthday. In Peru, the figure is 110 (Brown 1975:6).

In villages of the Ganges delta in Bangladesh, when summer rains flood rice-fields and roads, "children eat only once a day. Each year, this season generates a rash of funerals of infants and young children" (Brown 1975:3). Among the Iteso people of Uganda the month of May is called "the month when the children wait for food" because it is in these months:

"when the millet crop is growing and ripening ... that the spectre of malnutrition stalks the land. It is in these months that many children, weakened by malnourishment can die of illnesses which would hardly affect normal children" (McDowell 1975:28).

In these poor countries, where death certificates are issued "the death of pre-school children ... is generally attributed to measles, pneumonia, dysentery, or some other disease, but in fact these children are often victims of malnutrition" (Brown 1975:6). Nor is the impact of undernourishment limited to death during early years: "Recent experiments with monkeys have shown that severe malnutrition during formative years results in emotional problems of difficulty in adapting to change later on" (Brown 1975:6).

Hunger, malnutrition and child mortality are by no means the only forms of child maltreatment engendered by the world socioeconomic order. There are others, such as lack of proper education, lack of self-actualization, and insecurity. In Apa, Ghana, for instance, the coupling of ignorance with superstition has produced a curious type of medical maltreatment. According to Kaye (1962), "if a child refuses his meal it means he is feverish and so red pepper and ginger are ground and pushed down the rectum to make the child warm and promote an appetite. This medicine is very hot and painful so children try to avoid it as much as possible by eating whatever is given them" (1962:81).

Institutionalized maltreatment

At the second operational level, "non-societal" maltreatment subdivides into two broad categories: "deviant" and institutionalized ("non-deviant") maltreatment. "Deviant" maltreatment consists of those parental and other behaviours of adults towards children which a given culture considers as departure from approved child-rearing practices, and hence unacceptable. Institutionalized maltreatment consists of those practices sanctioned and approved by a given culture but which nonetheless have some detrimental effects on the child's well-being and development.

Institutionalized maltreatment, in most of the non-industrialized countries, falls into two distinct groupings.

27

1. Punitive maltreatment (Punishment)

In the words of Schmitt (1980), "disciplining children in painful ways or corporal punishment" is what is referred to here as punitive maltreatment. It is maltreatment intended by the perpetrator as a disciplinary measure. It consists of child-rearing practices which one group may view as acceptable and appropriate punishment but another regards as unacceptable and abusive. Commonest among these are physical punishment — caning, beating, spanking — and harsh punishment.

In general, child-rearing norms and values of most non-industrialized countries tend to favour physical punishment as a way of enforcing discipline. For instance, in his study of child-rearing practices in Nigeria, James Hake found that Northern Nigerian parents "believe that if one is too lenient in training a child he will bring misfortune to himself and his family. Therefore, 'spare the rod and spoil the child' becomes the dominant philosophy underlying the disciplinary methods of parents . . . As a result, corporal punishment is used quite freely on both boys and girls" (1972:39). According to him, 86.2% of the boys and 82.0% of the girls interviewed admitted that their parents or guardians used corporal punishment on them. Types of punishment included beating, whipping, denial of food, and restriction of free movement. However, he found sex differentiation in the pattern of punishment — male children are punished more by male parents or guardians and girls are punished more by their mothers (1972, Tables 58–61; pp. 90–91).

In the same vein, Kaye (1962) reported that in Tutu, Ghana, thumb-sucking is regarded as a bad habit which, if not curbed, may lead to gluttony. To stop it, "children are threatened, beaten, or their thumbs are cut and pepper rubbed in" (1962:75).

Toilet training is another child-rearing practice that attracts physical punishment in most non-industrialized countries. In Ghana, Kaye reports that a child who persists in wetting the bed after the age of five is subjected to a traditional punishment: "Early in the morning he is pulled out of bed, wrapped in his wet mat, smeared with clay or rubbed with stinging nettles, led to the sea or river accompanied by a crowd of jeering children and thrown in" (1962:91). The Igbo of Niger have similar shock treatments for bed-wetting. After repeated warnings, a dead snake is tied around the child's waist for some minutes. The trauma and shock which this experience produces serves to inhibit further bed-wetting.

2. Non-punitive customary practices

These are culturally sanctioned, societally approved practices, rites, ceremonies and customs which have no punitive motive but are in some way injurious to the child. In other words, such maltreatments are committed not in the name of child discipline but as customarily acceptable ways of living or doing things in that community. In the non-industrialized countries such maltreatments occur in various forms. They include:

Child marriage. Child marriage is a custom that is approved and practised in most Third World countries. Data from the Bangladesh 1981 census show that 7% of girls aged 10–14 and 65% of those aged 15–19 years were married; 75% of all girls in rural Bangladesh were married before the age of 20, compared with only 8% of teenage boys. "Not only are girls married much earlier, the age difference between husband and wife is also very wide" (Islam, 1985:8). Uchendu reports that "until it was legally abolished in 1956, child marriage was the most common way of acquiring rights in women. The Igbo girl was betrothed early, sometimes before she was a year old" (1965:50). In a recent study in Bangladesh, a respondent recalled that her grandmother "was engaged at the age of 40 days and went to the house of her father-in-law at the age of seven. Her husband was 18" (Islam, 1985:8).

The harmful effects of child marriage are too obvious to need recounting. It often generates mental stress in the child-wife. The great disparity in ages between husband and wife causes a generation gap, with the result that the child-wife often fails to respond to the husband's demands and expectations. In the words of Islam, "This has a serious effect on the psychology of the young wives, many of whom may suffer from mental depression and in extreme cases some even commit suicide" (1985:9). In addition, child marriage promotes high maternal mortality and, as studies have shown, "Children born of a teenage mother usually have low weight at birth, and are often undernourished" (Islam, 1985:9).

Child fostering (transfer). Child fostering — also referred to as child fosterage, child transfer, child exchange, child lending — has been defined as "the relocation or transfer of children from biological or natal homes to other homes where they are raised and cared for by foster parents" (Isiugo-Abanihe, 1985:53). The practice of child fostering is found in many non-industrialized countries. For instance, Ainsworth (1967) has reported its existence in Uganda, Uchendu (1965) in Nigeria, Keesing (1970) in Oceania, Rwason and Berggren (1973) in Haiti, Sanford (1975) in the West Indies. However, it is in West Africa that this practice appears most prevalent and highly developed. Here fostering starts early, in many cases even before the age of one, when the child is sent away, usually to the grandmother, to facilitate weaning. Under the impact of urbanization, this practice has taken on new dimensions: nowadays children are boarded out to not only blood relatives but also friends, acquaintances and even complete strangers. Further, it is not only the children of families that are in crisis or poor that are fostered out. Also, "both stable and unstable families, married and single mothers, healthy and handicapped parents, rural and urban homes, wealthy and poor parents" freely engage in this practice (Isiugo-Abanihe, 1985:56).

Five types of child fostering found in the non-industrialized countries have been identified (Isiugo-Abanihe, 1985):

(i) Kinship fostering, when children are sent to live with grandparents or other blood relations as an expression of traditional kinship obligations and mutual support.

(ii) Crisis fostering, when a child is taken away from its family as a child-welfare intervention measure. This happens when the natal family is facing such a crisis as divorce, separation, death of a spouse, becoming refugees, or physical disability (Obikeze and Mere, 1985:19).

(iii) Alliance/apprentice fostering, when fostering is used to establish and strengthen social, economic, political and religious alliances and bonds (Sinclair 1972). Isiugo-Abanihe (1985:57) recalls that in the Muslim cultures children, especially boys, are sent to live with influential religious leaders (mallams) to receive training and instruction in the Koran.

(iv) Educational fostering, when the purpose is to enable the child to receive formal education.

(v) Domestic fostering, when children are sent out to provide domestic and household services to the fostering family.

Fostering invariably entails removing the child from natural parents, from parental love and the ideal environment for its upbringing. This always creates psychological problems in later life. For one thing, a child denied parental love will be poorly equipped to give it as a parent. Where the foster-parent is not a relative of the child, the stage is well set for all sorts of disciplining maltreatment and neglect. Most of the time the foster-child is maltreated as much by the foster-parents as by their children, who may be of his own age or even younger.

Child pawning. Child pawning has been defined as "the practice of giving out a child as security for money borrowed or services rendered" (Obikeze, 1984:31). A pawned child is virtually stripped of all human dignity and freedom. He becomes very like a slave, with the main difference that whereas a slave is in perpetual bondage a pawn may be redeemed whenever the pawner can pay his debts.

The practice of pawning has been reported in many non-industrialized countries, such as India, Ghana and Nigeria. A recent study in Nigeria has shown that in each of 10 of the country's 19 states at least one person admitted to being aware of the occurrence of pawning within the previous five years (Obikeze, 1984:32). In Ghana, "A maternal uncle had also the right to pawn his sister's children to pay for clan debts" (Kaye, 1962:19).

Pawns, who are little better than slaves, may spend their whole childhood in the service of creditors — a situation which promotes the worst forms of dehumanization and abuse. Female pawns may be turned into wives or concubines if they are not redeemed by the time they attain maturity.

Caste system. Many Third-World societies have a system of stratification which sets a class of people apart and does not allow them to mix freely with persons outside their class. They are declared social outcasts and anyone interacting with them in unapproved ways is obliged to undergo purification. The Indian caste system is the best known and most developed but other varieties and modifications are found elsewhere. The "osu" (slaves of gods) system among the Igbo of Nigeria is a case in point (Obikeze 1984).

Although the caste system is now legally prohibited in these countries, informally and unofficially the descendants of such families continue to be regarded as "not-free-borns" and are despised, discriminated against and denied full citizenship status. Their children suffer a number of societal discriminations and deprivations. Quite early in the socialization process such children are made aware of their low social standing and this has serious psychological consequences for their personality development.

30

Maltreatment as deviant behaviour ("Deviant" maltreatment)

From a look at the analytical framework (Fig. I above) it may become obvious that much of what is treated in current literature on child maltreatment comes under this heading. Maltreatment of children as deviant behaviour embraces all acts and omissions of parents and other individuals and groups which do not conform with their communities' child-rearing norms and values. For analytical and diagnostic purposes, such deviant behaviour has been grouped into four broad types — child abuse, child neglect, child battering and child exploitation. Their various manifestations in the non-industrialized countries will now be discussed.

Child abuse. Child abuse as deviant behaviour occurs in four main categories:

(i) Physical abuse: Violence against children or physical child-abuse is probably the commonest form of child maltreatment in the non-industrialized countries. Its perpetrators include child-minders, siblings, teachers, religious leaders, peer groups, and others. Its basis lies in the culturally approved child-rearing norms of these countries. As Pfohl Stephen has put it, "the purposeful beating of the young has for centuries found legitimacy in the belief of its necessity for achieving disciplinary, educational or religious obedience" (1977:310).

In Nigeria, as in most other African countries, child socialization norms permit, and indeed enjoin, the use of the cane. In such cultures, child-beating becomes abusive only when it deviates from the approved patterns. For instance, among the Igbo of Nigeria, child-beating is considered physical abuse and therefore objectionable only "if it has a malicious intent; if it becomes a frequent occurrence; if it is severe; if bare fists or instruments other than the cane are used; and if the cane is too big (oversized) for the age and stature of the child" (Obikeze 1984). Apart from beating, other forms of physical abuse which occur in non-industrialized countries include burning, maiming, applying pepper or other hot substances to the eye or body, chaining and exposure to heat or cold.

(ii) Social abuse: Social abuse of children is manifested in the very low status accorded to children in most non-industrialized countries. Robert and Levine reported that among the Guisii-Nayansongo of Kenya, "before their initiation into adulthood, both boys and girls are considered to be of inferior status, (and) because of this lowly position, children are ordered about like servants and punished freely" (1963:151). In some communities children under the age of one are not counted as human beings. In addition, children suffer various kinds of social and legal discrimination on account of race, ethnicity or family status. Illegitimacy deserves special mention. This has to do with unequal rights of children born in wedlock and those born outside it; the latter may be labelled "illegitimate children", "hidden children", or "bastards" and are exposed to public disdain and even persecution (Veillard-Cybulska, 1975:33). In some countries, according to a UNICEF study, "incomplete registration of births, associated perhaps with a high rate of illegitimacy deprives a considerable number of children of important rights and social benefits to which they would otherwise be entitled under the law" (UNICEF, 1963:14).

(iii) Emotional abuse: Various patterns of emotional or psychological abuse of children are found in the non-industrialized countries. It may take the form of

31

nagging, scolding, ridicule, scapegoating, etc. Such acts if sustained tend to make the child nervous, lose self-confidence, and develop aggressive or withdrawal tendencies. The importance attached to ridicule, a form of psychological abuse, in the African culture is reflected in the following statement of Professor T. A. Lambo:

> A factor worth mentioning in the socialization of Nigerian children is that of ridicule which is a very potent social control. Ridicule is a formidable (and dangerous) weapon in the hands of those who seem to mould the child to a traditional pattern of life. (1969:69).

(iv) Sexual and drug abuse: Sexual abuse and drug abuse are other forms of child abuse found in both industrialized and non-industrialized countries. However, the particularly private nature of these offences is reflected in the paucity of documentary evidence about them in the developing countries.

Child neglect. Neglect of children is widespread in the non-industrialized countries. Daily activities are generally woven around adult-centred pursuits and in the heat of these activities the welfare of children tends to be forgotten or, at best, given second place. Child neglect may occur with regard to nurture, health, clothing, education, etc. In Nigeria some market women and traders leave their homes before dawn and return late at night, leaving their teenage children in the care of housemaids and older siblings. In Haiti, Matheson (1975) observed similar neglect of children: babies and young children in Haiti are left with older sisters and other women when the mother goes out to work. "The result is that many babies receive a very irregular supply of breast milk, and when the mother is away from home the infant often goes hungry or is given unsuitable food as substitutes" (1975:24). Similarly, in Bompata (Asante) Ghana, Kaye reports that "it is very common to see little children aged between three and five whose parents have left them at home without any proper arrangements having been made for their feeding" (1962:80). Educational neglect of children is also very common, particularly among the Fulani pastoralists in West Africa and other migrant groups.

Child battering. As indicated earlier, child battering differs from physical child abuse only in severity. Earlier observations on physical abuse are therefore equally applicable here.

Child exploitation. A study carried out in Nigeria by the author showed that exploitation of the child for economic gain ranked highest among the various forms of child maltreatment mentioned by the respondents (Obikeze 1984, Table 1). Child exploitation occurs in diverse forms and may be perpetrated by parents, foster-parents, employers, master tradesmen and guardians.

To some extent, child exploitation in the non-industrialized countries has its base in their child-rearing norms, which prescribe that within the household children should be assigned and made to carry out some domestic activities suitable to their age, sex and physical ability. Traditionally, such activities serve to socialize the young into future adult roles. They are also a source of pride, self-esteem and independence for children, while at the same time providing an important supplement to the family income. However, this cultural provision

32

has been quite often abused, giving rise to various forms of economic exploitation of children. The following illustrations of certain manifestations of child exploitation are drawn essentially from the Nigerian scene. Positions in which Nigerian children are most frequently exploited include the following:

a) *As domestic servants:* In many Nigerian homes, particularly in the cities and towns, school-age children are employed, occasionally full-time, as house-servants, baby-sitters or child-minders. At times such servants receive paltry monthly allowances or must content themselves with board and lodging. In the villages such domestic servants, and even the biological children, work on the land or in handicrafts for the family's benefit. The exploitative, and therefore abusive, nature of these activities does not lie in the amount of unpaid-for wealth produced, but rather in that they are often too strenuous and take up the time that should be used for the child's education and for play.

b) *As street beggars:* In Nigeria, as in many other countries in Africa and Asia, it is common to see in the streets children of all ages, bowls in hand, begging for alms. They may be accompanied by adults or may be sent by their adult exploiters — parents, foster-parents, or Koranic teachers (mallams). According to Eraedu, "children are seen standing or sitting under the sun and feeling the excruciating pain of hunger, while they beg for alms" (1982:22). Yet, these children carry on their assignments, patiently, obediently and conscientiously, day by day; and at the end of each day they turn in the proceeds to the parent or mallam so as to earn that days' meal (Obikeze 1984).

c) *As child prostitutes:* Studies have shown that elderly prostitutes often use children left in their care as baits to attract customers. At times such women organize brothels where they employ school drop-outs and other delinquent children for purposes of making money.

d) *As hawkers:* In many countries of West Africa, parents and guardians frequently exploit children by using them as hawkers and street sales-boys and sales-girls. "In the market places, in the motor parks, and along busy streets, under the scorching heat of the sun, children are seen carrying baskets full of wares, shouting at the top of their voices to attract the attention of interested buyers" (Obikeze, 1984, Eraedu 1982). For some of the children hawking or street trading is a full-time occupation, leaving no time for schooling or play. For others who manage to attend school, hawking starts as soon as school is over and continues late into the night.

e) *As apprentices:* Traditionally in Nigeria, formal training in one of the specialized occupations takes place as a period of apprenticeship. Nowadays, this principle is being manipulated to exploit children. The master insists on an apprenticeship of, say, five years for a job that would easily be learnt in two and a half to three years. The result is that the child spends the last two years rendering free service to the master. This means that if a workman has, say, seven apprentices he will eventually have a work-force of five or more persons working for him daily, free of charge for two or more years. In addition, at the end of each day's work, the apprentice renders domestic services to the master's household.

f) *As bus conductors:* A special group of exploited children which Eraedu highlighted in his study of Lagos, Nigeria, is bus conductors or bus attendants. Eraedu reported that to win passengers these bus-boys are made to "jump off moving vehicles as bus stops are approached" and begin sing-songs with names of bus stops or the bus routes that they operate (Eraedu, 1982). In return, the boys are given food, board (at times) and some pocket money.

These by no means exhaust the ways in which children are economically exploited in non-industrialized societies, but it is hoped that the examples given are enough to sensitize world opinion to the seriousness of the problem.

Summary and Conclusion

In this paper, I have tried to do two things: first, to provide a common classification and standardized operational definition of a variety of terms and concepts currently in use in the field of child maltreatment; and second, to develop a comprehensive analytical framework for describing the various dimensions of the phenomenon of child maltreatment as it is manifested in non-industrialized countries. Although the analytical framework presented in this paper has been developed with the non-industrialized world in mind, it is equally applicable to the industrialized countries and in this respect it provides a scheme for comparison of patterns of child maltreatment in the two world orders.

Thus if, for instance, we take the first operational level, the global level (Fig. I), it becomes apparent that societal maltreatment is generated by such factors as, in the non-industrialized countries, underdevelopment, inequality, poverty, ignorance, superstition, ethnicity, and racism, and, in the industrialized countries, unemployment, urban overcrowding, family disorganization, and alienation.

At the cultural level (Level II), it is apparent that institutionalized maltreatment is more prevalent and plays a more significant role in the non-industrialized than in the industrialized countries. Indeed, it appears that as a country advances in industrialization and modernization the patterns of child maltreatment change from institutionalized to "deviant" individualized forms.

The intellectual community is called upon to explore further the latent potential of this analytical framework.

References

[1]. Ainsworth, M.D.S. *Infancy in Uganda.* Baltimore, the Johns Hopkins University Press, 1967.

[2] Braden, A. Adopting the abused child: love is not enough. *Social casework,* Vol. 62, No. 6, 1981.

[3] Brown, R. Death at an early age. *UNICEF NEWS,* 85, No. 3, 1975.

[4] Cantwell, N. Parental physical violence towards children. *Assignment children,* Vol. 47, 1979.

[5] Eraedu, The Nigerian child: a victim of exploitation. *The Sunday Times,* November 14, 1982.

[6] Gil, G. *Violence against children.* Cambridge, Mass., Harvard University Press, 1970.

[7] Giovannoni, J.M. Parental mistreatment: perpetrators and victims. *Journal of marriage and family,* Vol. 33 (1971).

[8] Hake, J.M. *Child-rearing practices in Northern Nigeria.* Ibadan University Press, 1972.

[9] Hobcraft, J. WFS: a final assessment. *People,* Vol. 12 (3) (1985).

[10] Isiugo-Abanihe, U.C. Child fosterage in West Africa. *Population and development review,* 11 (1) (1985).
[11] Islam, M. Child wives of Bangladesh *People,* 12 (3) 1985.
[12] Kaye, B. *Bringing up children in Ghana.* London, George Allen and Unwin, 1962.
[13] Keesing, R. Kwaio fosterage. *American anthropologist,* 72 (1970).
[14] Kempe, H.C. and Helfer, R.E. (eds.), *The battered child.* Chicago, University of Chicago Press, 1980.
[15] Lambo, T.A. The Child and the mother-child relationship in major cultures of Africa. *Assignment children,* 10 (1979).
[16] Matheson, A. The grim facts of life in Haiti. *UNICEF NEWS,* 85 (3) 1975.
[17] McDowell, J. The month when the children wait for food, *UNICEF NEWS,* 85 (3) 1975.
[18] Obikeze, D.S. Perspectives on child abuse in Nigeria. *International child welfare review* 63 (1984).
[19] Obikeze, D.C. and Mere, A.A. *Children and the Nigerian civil war.* Nsukka, University of Nigeria Press, 1985.
[20] Pfohl, S.J. The discovery of child abuse. *Social problems,* 24 (3) 1977.
[21] Rawson, I.G. and Berggen, G. Family structure, child location and nutritional diseases in rural Haiti. *Environmental child health, 19 (3) 1973.*
[22] Reubens, E.P. *Planning for children and youth within national development planning.* Geneva, UN Research Institute for Social Development and United Nations Children's Fund, 1967.
[23] Robert A. and Levine B. Nyansongo, a Guisii community in Kenya. *Six cultures,* B. Whiting (ed.), New York, John Wiley, 1963.
[24] Sanford, M. To be treated as a child of the home: Black Carib child-lending in British West Indian society. *Socialization and communication in primary groups,* T.R. Williams (ed.), The Hague, Mouton, 1975.
[25] Schmitt, D. Battered child syndrome. *Current pediatric diagnosis and treatment,* H.C. Kemp et al. (eds.). Los Altos, California Lange Medical Publications, 1980.
[26] Sinclair, J. Educational assistance, kinship, and the social structure in Sierra Leone. *African research bulletin,* 2 (3), 1972.
[27] Sweet, J.J. and Resick, P.A. The maltreatment of children: a review of theories and research. *Journal of social issues,* 35 (2) 1979.
[28] Uchendu, V.C. *The Igbo of South-East Nigeria.* New York, Holt, Rinehart and Winston, 1965.
[29] United Nations Childrens Fund (UNICEF), *Children of the developing countries.* London, Thomas Nelson & Sons Ltd., 1963.
[30] Veillard-Cybulska, H. The legal welfare of children in a disturbed family situation. *International child welfare review,* 27 (1975).

35

DISCUSSION

Carballo: First let me congratulate both speakers for two excellent presentations, which take us well on the road to reaching the goal of this conference. I was intrigued by the fact that, on the one hand, Dr Krugman suggested that we not try to seek definitions, and, on the other, Dr Obikeze not only went to great length to seek definitions but also gave us a very useful analytical model. If, as Dr. Obikeze suggests in his diagram, we take the fact that what we are dealing with is the maltreated child as the end-result, would Dr Krugman not agree that, unless we can devise certain types of definitions, or at least promote a discussion at a public-health level about the different forms of child treatment we shall not be able to determine what we should or should not do, what are the inappropriate or appropriate entry-points into different situations. You talk, for example, about non-organic failure to thrive, a subject which I think would intrigue anyone from a public-health point of view, and in Dr Obikeze's schema he refers to institutionalized maltreatment. I think there are situations where non-organic failure to thrive has become a well-established institutionalized form of maltreatment. It may not be open to the same type of care or intervention that perhaps some of the deviant maltreatment you are seeing in your clinic settings is, but I think that unless we can try to define them in this way we shall not be able to deal with the problem as we should.

Morrow: My question to Dr Obikeze concerns the one problem that was not mentioned in your discussion — what are his views on the problem of child or baby circumcision, particularly of circumcision of girls in Africa and in the Arab world? I think this is a problem that the medical and the nursing professions have not really tackled, and I hope that during this conference it will be touched upon.

Gellhorn: My question is addressed to Dr Krugman and also to the Chairman. In 1973 in New York State the New York State Child Protective Services Act was enacted, which made reporting of child abuse and neglect a reportable disease. When it was first enacted there were 30,000 reports involving 60,000 children. Year by year this has increased, and in 1984 there were 81,000 reports involving 135,000 children. The reports were made to the Department of Social Services or the Department of Health in the State, and were for purposes of investigating and providing rehabilitative and preventive services. In discussing with other members of the conference I found that reporting was not done in other countries on the grounds that it would be an invasion of privacy and might be counter-productive. Now, what is the correct answer?

Ramazanoglu: My first question, directed to Dr Krugman, concerns the practical side of the problem. What would be your advice to the general practitioners and paediatricians working in their private offices? Should they evaluate and treat the case themselves or should they think of the complexity and many other different aspects of the problem and send the child to the nearest medical centre where there is a special team responsible for child abuse? My second question is directed to both Dr Krugman and Dr Obikeze. Is there any correlation between child abuse and the number of children in the family?

Dogramaci: I think this brings up the very important matter of the professional secret. We have taken an oath not to reveal anything without the parents' permission. But what if a legal case comes up — there have been court cases a couple of years back in Britain? Usually parents have nothing against reporting a notifiable disease, because it is law, but if they have committed some sort of a crime, broken a bone, are we allowed to report against their wishes? I think this may come up during the group discussions.

Adadevoh: I congratulate Dr Obikeze for a good general outline of the subject, which should permit us during the week to have a meaningful global dialogue with some clarity, bearing in mind differences that can occur here and there. The various definitions which he has given us should guide us over some of these differences. I realize that Dr Krugman, in advising us not to get into the nitty-gritty of defining abuse and neglect, was very conscious of the differences which can occur from place to place. I say this because during the next two days I am certain that we are going to find a number of woolly areas which will require some give and take in order to come to a consensus, but let me address one or two issues that came from your paper. One is the question of emotional abuse. We have to be careful here who decides. When I looked at your slide, and if I tested myself on some of those issues you raised and also some of what Dr Obikeze mentioned, I wonder whether I can say that I have not been abusing my children. One would like to know when taking a questionnaire amongst parents, feeding some of this information to them in various cultures. We have to be a little conscious also in not wanting to rapidly bring sociocultural or other changes into environments which we do not know about. I was tempted to ask about circumcision myself, but I do not want to get bogged down by the arguments for and against circumcision, which have been many times brandished from various parts of the world. As to what happens in some of the cultural settings in Africa, I think we have to wait until those things change gradually. What I am saying in effect is that we have to realize that we are dealing with a subject where physical abuse, including sexual abuse and other forms, which are clearly visible and quantifiable, are the ones we can really bite. There will be many other areas which will provide us with some understanding only if we realize that this is a changing phenomenon.

Lesnik Oberstein: It is true that if you view abuse acts behaviouristically, then abuse is what a culture defines as abuse — and the definition of abuse remains culture-specific. But if you take into account the meaning of an act for the child — as Dr Krugman suggested — then it is possible to arrive at a cross-cultural definition of abuse. Any act that harms a child within a certain culture, social and class context is abuse. For example, if in a certain culture it is believed that in order to grow up to be a self-reliant adult a child must be caned ten times when he becomes ten years old, and the child shares this belief, the culture won't regard the caning as abuse — and neither will the child. But if an American middle-class father canes his 10-year-old child ten times because the child accidentally spilled a glass of water, the child will experience it as abuse — and it will be abuse. One caning constitutes abuse and the other not because the meaning of the act for the child is different in the two cultural contexts. To make a very long story short, it seems that when you look at abuse behaviouristically, then indeed you are culture-locked. But if you look at the meaning for the child of the act being carried out, then it is possible to arrive at a cross-cultural definition of child abuse.

Browne: I would like to pick up Dr Krugman's comment that we have 90% of the knowledge we need to be able to recognize sexual abuse. Certainly we don't have 100% knowledge to identify abusing parents and that is why prevention and treatment programmes are still in their infancy. For example, in Surrey, where I work, 15% of parents show fewer than four of those typical characteristics, and therefore what I would like to know is what leads parents who don't show these typical characteristics to abuse the children. I think therefore we need — I would like to emphasize the previous comment — we need adequate, internationally-adopted definitions because the trouble with a lot of American work is heterogeneous samples where they probably haven't defined their sample into physical abusers, sexual abusers, and neglecters, and until we do that the psychosocial problems of each of those types of individuals cannot be adequately looked at and treatment programmes adequately assessed.

Goodwin: Does Dr Krugman have any ideas about what the mediator might be between the unemployment rate which he indicated and the reported rate of child abuse? Could it be that there might be a mediating factor such as poverty and how does that act? Would he care to make any observations about that? Secondly, would he like to give some examples of the primary prevention programmes — I hope that there are primary prevention programmes for child abuse. Lastly, I wonder whether Dr Obikeze would like to comment on whether any of those primary prevention programmes would seem to be appropriate to the sort of child abuse he was describing. And, I would like to put a word in for us all to note the frequency with which we have already heard today the term "disease", "reported disease", and we have heard the observation that child abuse is primarily a medical problem. I would ask us all to think whether in fact that is the right way to deal with a problem which already, from our two doctors we have heard, clearly has social and cultural aspects.

Dogramaci: We will now return to our speakers to respond to some of these questions. Nobody has asked what we should do to stop war, armed conflicts and terrorism. I think this is again a very important cause not only of child abuse but also of population abuse. I think perhaps the Big Powers will decide that.

Krugman: Let me explain better what I meant by not defining abuse and why I said it. Clearly, there are definitions, and, clearly, we arrive at them in different ways, and I suppose what I was saying was that, where we get into trouble in a group either in a community or in a country, or in a meeting, is never on certain parts of the spectrum of abuse or neglect but in the middle. Dr Obikeze asked what the difference is between discipline and abuse. Well, we could argue that forever. That's where our government spent a lot of money to not much end, in my opinion. If a society or a group of professionals considers what it is that all agree on, they have no trouble agreeing that when an infant is shaken to death, beaten to death, burned to death, or starved to death, this is abuse. Now if we begin with that definition and work on that as a country or a society or a world body, and we try to eliminate all murder, all shaking, all forms of physical abuse, then the issue of whether spanking is abuse will become a little easier to deal with. It makes no sense in my society to say that we must right now outlaw spanking when we still have 5,000 children a year who are being beaten, shaken to death, or who disappear and are murdered, and we are not taking swift action in that regard. I think we need to work at both ends. I am willing to stand up and say I don't believe in corporal punishment and we ought to eliminate it, but, politically, I know that before a law will be passed in the United States to outlaw corporal punishment we had better eliminate shakings, murders, burnings and other things that everyone does agree on. So that is what I meant by saying that we shouldn't define it. I don't want us to spend time on a grey area where we can't agree. What we should do and that is what Dr Lesnik Oberstein in essence pointed out, is to try to define those areas where we can all agree. If we work from that, the task will be easier.

Dr Gellhorn discussed the issue of reporting, that it's done in the United States, not in other countries, and that it's an invasion of privacy. Time will tell whether that approach is correct. There is no doubt that mandatory reporting by professionals in the United States has led to fixing of responsibility for the child protective service system on our departments of social services. Before mandatory reporting it was too easy for everybody to say "that's not my problem", and, practically speaking, physicians and social workers and others have had that problem. I have seen cases and been called about cases from all over the world where there isn't a reporting system. Children fall through the cracks and everybody says "it's their problem". The physicians say it's the social workers' fault, the social workers say it is the fault of the police, the police say it's the courts' fault, the courts say it's the doctors', and everybody points to everybody else and meanwhile you have a dead child. We may not have a perfect system but at least we know where the responsibility lies, and I think that is an important step. As far as invasion of privacy goes, I will quote from Dr Kempe. He said no child ever died of a social worker's evaluation but that many died because we didn't get a report. I believe he was right.

The advice we should give to paediatricians and general practitioners is that physicians should not try to handle this alone, and it gets back to the comment over here which says "whose problem is this"? Abuse and neglect is not a medical or a social or a legal problem: it is a child's problem and a family's problem, and it requires all professionals in medicine, law, social work and the legal system to work together. At our hospital, the core team is the group that works with these cases every day — a physician, a social worker and a coordinator. We need a coordinator because we have 400 cases a year and six counties with which we have to deal. The consultative team meets every week and includes an attorney, an adult psychiatrist, a nurse, a psychologist, a developmental specialist and a child psychiatrist. They meet with the paediatrician and the social worker and the coordinator and they discuss cases week after week. Some of them have been doing it for 25 years, reviewing cases every week, and they have extensive clinical experience in dealing with these cases and the families and the system. Outside are the individuals for each family and each case: a county attorney, a teacher, a foster-parent, a guardian, a mental health therapist, a police officer, an intake social worker, a family health public nurse, a family physician — each one case-specific. So my advice is that you need centres of excellence, you need individuals — this is a consultative service just as we have consultative services and centres where we send premature infants at 800 or 1,000 grams. We don't expect general physicians or general paediatricians to be able to care for a 1,000 gram baby with complex heart disease. We send those babies to a centre where there are experts. I think the same approach should be with child abuse. One of the things we have to do better is to disseminate that expertise and regionalize the confidential doctor system. The Netherlands is a good example of developing that type of expertise and centralizing it. I don't care what the system is, there needs to be experts.

Is there a correlation between child abuse and neglect and numbers of children in a family? The answer is yes and no. Clearly, there are families where one child is targetted and many children or other children in the family do fine. That is true of neglect, especially of deprivation dwarfism, and it's true of physical abuse. There are other families that are so disorganized, or so abusive, that all children are abused and neglected. Each case needs to be looked at individually.

With regard to emotional abuse and who decides — I can tell you very honestly that I have, at times, been emotionally abusive to some of my children — I have four — to all of them at one time or another. There have been times when I felt like being physically abusive — when they have angered me, and I have felt like picking them up and throwing them against the wall — and each of them knows that, and each of them knows that I haven't done it because I have recognized that, when I have felt like doing it, it was time to turn to my wonderful wife and say "you take them, I have had it!" Now I submit that that is what separates abusive parents from non-abusive parents, and that there are other influences such as drugs and alcohol, and stresses such as unemployment, that may erode an adult's self-esteem. Maybe put them in contact with a child for many more hours during a day than when they are working, maybe because it is related to poverty, maybe because it is related to time. I don't know what the full answer is as regards unemployment, and why we see an increase; there are many abused children where there is full employment in the family, and so it is not just poverty.

As to who decides whether something is abusive, it is in my view the child. If the child feels it's abusive, then it is abusive, and that is really what we are trying to look at — how the child manifests the behaviour, what is the reaction of children to certain acts that we as individuals or society do.

Obikeze: The last speaker has answered a number of the questions that relate to my paper. However, on the issue of definitions, I want to say that it is important, indeed necessary, for the growth of knowledge, for the growth of any science. We need to define, we need to classify, the terms we use; otherwise terms will be used anyhow and different persons may use the same terms or words to mean different things in different contexts. Such a situation does not make for scientific progress. Thus it is necessary that at a certain point in the development of this discipline we should come to an agreement to reserve certain meanings to specific terms, and thereafter everyone working in the field comes to know it to be so, to accept it to be so, and to use it in subsequent discussions. In this way, research can progress.

In my paper, what I have done with regard to classification is to acknowledge and make allowance for the existence of cultural differences. Thus when I classify some forms of child maltreatment as belonging to "institutionalized" or "non-deviant" types I mean that each cultural area or society will identify the prevailing forms of maltreatment that fall into the categories. For instance, in cultures where child marriage is prevalent, it falls under this category. In cultures where the practice is not institutionalized it falls into a different category.

As regards emotional abuse — what constitutes emotional abuse? I feel that it is for scientists and practitioners operating in a given cultural milieu to determine what constitutes emotional abuse in that area. With regard to whether scolding a child constitutes emotional abuse, I would disagree with the last speaker, who held that it is the child who should determine whether and when it becomes abusive. I think that it is society, the normative codes of the society in question, that will determine this. For instance, a father can become very angry at a child and scold him. The child, despite his misbehaviour, may not like being scolded, but I do not think it right to declare the father's action abusive simply because the child feels so. However, it becomes abusive if the act of scolding persists and becomes a pattern of interaction, which, of course, the society does not approve of.

With regard to female circumcision, although it was not specifically mentioned in my paper it is adequately provided for in the schema — it will be one of the institutionalized forms of maltreatment if it is proven that the practice is injurious to the child's health. In other words, and bearing in mind Professor Adadevoh's comments on this issue, the inclusion of female circumcision as a form of maltreatment is dependent upon evidence from the medical profession.

Also, there is the question of some correlation between the number of children in the family (family size) and the incidence of child abuse. I think that it depends on individual parents, their personal characteristics. A large number of children may predispose to such other factors as poverty and scarcity of resources but, just as not all parents of large families become abusive, not all abusive parents are parents of large families.

Dogramaci: I think the main question was female circumcision and you say it is medical. Perhaps Dr Petros-Barvazian could tell us that many hundreds of female babies die — I don't think it is anywhere medically condoned.

Krugman: I neglected to answer the question about prevention and to clarify the comment that I said we have 90% of the knowlege we need to have and yet 15% of the families only showed four of the characteristics that I showed on the slide. Let me point out that those are the characteristics we use to differentiate accidental from non-accidental injury. They are not parental characteristics *per se*. You can have a whole list of psychological characteristics of parents, including low self-esteem and other types of issues that I did not include. In our prevention programmes we can recognize who is at risk for abuse and neglect. We know that if we support those at risk of physical abuse and neglect with home visitors, or with nurturing types of outreach mothers, we can reduce substantially severe physical abuse. We don't turn those parents into the warmest, kindest, most wonderful, human beings you ever met, but we do prevent them from severely harming their children.

Sexual abuse prevention remains to be seen. We need better data as to whether we are actually preventing sexual abuse, or whether we are using those programmes to better identify children who have already been sexually abused.

Adadevoh: I thought I should just protect the question which we heard — the question on circumcision. It might have been implied that it was female circumcision, but my interjection, and Dr Obikeze's, referred to circumcision generally. If it is female circumcision then I repeat the plea I made earlier on, to leave the environment to develop the attitude to decide to discontinue. What I have noticed in the past is that all the movements to try to stop circumcision in Africa have generated resistance rather than success. As to whether it is harmful or not, it depends on what exactly you are doing. I think we don't want to get involved in that now.

Petros-Barvazian: I agree with the speaker before me that this issue has been discussed at length. Female circumcision in different sociocultural settings, for the most part and in the circumstances in which it is carried out, is definitely harmful to the child's immediate health and we know that it causes complications during childbirth and the rest. From the purely medical point of view then, it is obvious. But the important thing is how various countries themselves are trying to tackle the issue. To put it into context — what are the harmful practices affecting the health of women and children, and what are the traditionally beneficial practices affecting the health of mothers and children? Traditional practices are not always harmful. This is an issue one has to keep in mind and within each culture try to tackle by whatever possible education of the public, the professionals and so on. We in WHO, in these issues of traditional practices affecting health, have taken them up and worked with countries at their request to study them and to begin to take some action to deal with the problem.

Dogramaci: Dr Obikeze, do you want to make a comment at this stage in response to what has been said? You said it has to be approved medically, and apparently for males circumcision is no problem provided it is done under hygienic conditions by a competent circumciser. There is not always a surgeon to do this. Rabbis do it in many places under sterile conditions. But regarding female circumcision I doubt whether there is any ground to justify it.

Obikeze: My comment is that the inclusion of this in any part of a schema would depend on the culture concerned. If, as mentioned, a society is not quite clear whether this is harmful, then once this society is satisfied that it is harmful it comes under institutionalized child abuse. It is for each society to decide where to include it in its schema.

42

SPECIFIC ASPECTS
OF THE PROBLEM

PHYSICAL ABUSE AND NEGLECT OF CHILDREN IN THE FAMILY: A REVIEW OF PSYCHOSOCIAL FACTORS

Brian Bell*

INTRODUCTION

Estimates suggest that each year in the United States of America as many as 2,000 children may die as a consequence of child abuse and neglect. During 1980 in North America, 999 children below the age of 14 years died as a result of 'homicide and injury purposely inflicted by other persons' (WHO, 1984). Another source states as a conservative estimate that each year in the United Kingdom over 100 babies are battered to death by their parents or guardians and over 8,000 children suffer "non-accidental injuries" (Kellmer-Pringle, 1980). These figures refer to reported and registered cases of abuse and neglect. How many more children undergo attempted strangulation, unsuccessful poisonings, enforced imprisonment, starvation, excessive and repeated corporal punishment, and emotional deprivation — the list is not exhaustive — remains a conjecture. The final figure may well be in hundreds of thousands.

That cruel and unjust treatment of children is not only a twentieth-century phenomenon is shown by historical evidence. More often than not, maltreatment of children has been deliberately employed in the pursuit of some individual or collective ideology. Jobling (1978) provides the following illustration from the fifteenth century, where a mother writes of her attempts to persuade her young and recalcitrant daughter to marry an elderly widower: "She hath since Easter the most part been beaten once in a week or twice, or sometimes twice in one day, and her head broken in two or three places".

Four hundred years later, in an age of burgeoning social concern, the reports of the Children's Employment Commissions in Victorian England show that Boards of Guardians were apprenticing boys of six years of age to coal-miners. The recorded experiences of one boy are probably not unrepresentative: having been "beaten by his master and had coals thrown at him", he slept in disused mine workings and ate candles to stay alive (Thompson, 1968). At the same time the mother of John Wesley, the religious reformer, was writing to her son on the topic of child care and advised, "Break their wills betimes; begin this great work before they can run alone, before they can speak plain, or perhaps speak at all . . . make him do as he is bid, if you whip him ten times running to effect it" (Jobling, 1978). Those who require further examples are recommended to consult recent articles by Jobling (1978) and Radbill (1980).

What in essence characterizes the second half of this century, however, is not

---

* Professor, Faculty of Community and Social Studies, Newcastle upon Tyne Polytechnic, Northumberland Building, Northumberland Road, Newcastle upon Tyne NE1 8ST, England

just the rediscovery of the 'battered child' (Kempe et al., 1962) or an academic realization that child cruelty does not belong to the historical archives, but rather the search for an explanation of cause and effect, and for ways and means of prediction and prevention.

What, then, may one ask, is the relevance of historical illustrations such as these? Even cursory reflection suggests that they may provide clues not only to an aetiology of abuse but also to avenues of prevention. Much effort, laudable in itself, and resources have been given over to the portrayal of child abuse and neglect as a medical phenomenon; only more recently have researchers established that child maltreatment is rooted in wider social processes, some of which are yet only partially understood. This lesson, we maintain, was long evident in the historical accounts described earlier — the expression of parental authority through physical violence, the concept of the child as a chattel of society to be exploited for economic purposes, and the inculcation of given moralities by the severe and authoritarian use of force.

A consideration of much research over the last two decades leaves the suspicion that many continue to hope that the social-process hypothesis will prove faulty and that some other elusive but as yet undiscovered factor will emerge to save us from having to reach what may be painful conclusions about cause and prevention. Sweet and Resick (1979) conclude that even if factors such as poverty and violence are fundamental causes of abuse nothing can be done about them. In their view, abuse results from modelling of inappropriate parental behaviour: social forces which act to establish, maintain and reinforce this behaviour are either disregarded or dismissed as being either intractable or insoluble. 'Purist' approaches which conceptualize child abuse as a phenomenon in its own right and consequently seek to determine a psychological 'cause' and an attendant 'cure' obscure the fact that, first and foremost, child abuse and neglect are social phenomena. In contrast, the social-phenomena approach does not deny the importance of biological or psychological factors but rather seeks to incorporate them within a wider conceptual framework.

This paper provides a survey of some recent psychological and sociological research into abuse and neglect. A strict division is not drawn between the two manifestations of maltreatment: physical injury and physical neglect. However, the majority of studies quoted deal with physical abuse or non-accidental injury. The problem of definition has received particular attention in the literature (cf. Gelles and Cornell, 1983): for present purposes, no major distinction is made between the 'classical' 1962 definition of Kempe (where diagnosable medical and physical symptoms are present) and the probabilistic definition (Straus et al., 1980), which includes a wider range of violent behaviour and its consequences.

Problems of definition are discussed further in the section dealing with incidence. This may be omitted by those who wish to proceed directly to an account, necessarily selective, of some empirical research on putative psychological and sociological factors in abuse. A brief review of some findings on the sequelæ of abuse again raises methodological issues, while the remaining sections deal with some aspects of prediction and prevention. The emphasis throughout is to refer to studies and work from the last 10 years or so.

For those who wish to delve back further, and indeed for those whose main concern is for treatment studies (which are not covered here in any systematic detail), a comprehensive review by Parke and Collmer (1975) will prove useful. Those who assume that the psycho-analytic aspects of abuse and neglect have been deliberately omitted are correct in their assumption: an earlier article by Steele (1970) deals with this area of concern.

INCIDENCE OF CHILD ABUSE

A major consequence of the lack of any unitary definition of child abuse and neglect is the wide variation in estimates of its incidence. Some researchers present data which are based on only severe cases of physical abuse (Baldwin and Oliver, 1975); others include a wider-ranging spectrum of abuse and include, for example, poisoning and drug overdosing, sexual abuse and failure to thrive (Creighton, 1979; Smith and Deasy, 1977). The incidence rates for non-Western societies are subject to this definitional problem to an even greater degree, where only Western researchers may consider acts such as initiation rites and other forms of 'ritualised punishment' (Field, 1983). to be abuse *per se.*

National and international incidence

Incidence rates are drawn from a variety of sources, which include national surveys (Gil, 1970), central reporting registers (Creighton, 1979; Gonzalez-Pardo and Thomas, 1977) and compilation of newspaper accounts (De Francis, 1983). Many estimates of incidence rates are extrapolations from 'opportunistic' case-studies or representative surveys (Straus et al. 1980). Nevertheless, over the last decade or so, estimates of incidence rates have tended to be revised upwards, reflecting in part a greater awareness of the problem by health-care and social-service professionals as well as an improvement in monitoring and reporting procedures. It would be as well to note that significant fluctuations in incidence rates occur over time: for example, recent data from the United Kingdom, compiled by the National Society for the Prevention of Cruelty to Children (NSPCC) (1985), indicate a decrease in fatal cases but a rise of some 11% in non-specific abuse over a one-year period. One study (Pieterse, 1977) reported an (unexplained) increase in the number of reported cases during the spring and autumn months.

One of the first national surveys of child abuse was carried out by Gil (1970) in the U.S.A. — in this it was estimated that the upper limits of child abuse would be between 2.5 and 4.0 million cases annually, equal to incidence rates of some 13 to 21 per 1000 population. Light (1973) subsequently revised these rates downwards by a factor of 10. A household survey (Gelles, 1978) suggested that between 1.5 and 2 million children are at risk for serious physical injury each year in the U.S.A. Data on incidence rates in the United Kingdom evidence similar variations: these range from high levels of between 75 and 93 per million (Hall, 1972: Smith and Hanson, 1974) to levels half these in other studies (Baldwin and Oliver, 1975). It is important to note that these incidence figures are based on extrapolations from data derived in a variety of settings, which differ even on a national basis both socioeconomically and geographically.

Accordingly, any comparison on an international basis of incidence rates is necessarily complicated by any or all of the factors which make intra-national comparisons of rates so suspect. Some rates are given here for illustrative purposes.

Smith and Deasy (1977) reported that child abuse, in a variety of forms, accounts for 1 in 700 childhood admissions to hospital in Ireland (an unexpectedly high frequency of abused twins was found in this study). In Japan, where child guidance clinics are required by law to report abuse cases, Ikeda (1982) suggests a figure of 2,000 severe cases annually. Estimates for Israel range from a low of 3,000 cases annually to a high of 10,000 (Brodie, 1982). Tauber et al. (1977) using current US estimates predicted 3,000–5,000 cases annually for Italy. Fergusson et al. (1972) reported an incidence rate of 0.26 per 1,000 children in New Zealand, with a reminder that the rate was likely to be higher among the Maori population. Dubanoski and Snyder (1980) found differential rates for Japanese Americans and Samoan Americans in Hawaii — the ratio of abuse to neglect for Japanese was 1:3 but for Samoans it was reversed (3:1). Zenz (1978) using police statistics in the Federal Republic of Germany for 1975 reports a rate of 0.11 per 1,000, a rate considered to be very much an underestimate owing to many cases not being reported to the authorities.

In contrast, Vesterdal (1977) considered that missed cases in Denmark would likely be low, given the extensive national social-welfare system, and gave an incidence of 0.035 per 1,000 for Greater Copenhagen. In Sweden, where some 500 to 600 cases of suspected abuse are reported each year to child welfare centres, about 10 children a year require inpatient treatment — this corresponds to an approximate incidence rate for severe injury of only 0.026 per 1,000 children.

In Third World countries estimates of the incidence of child abuse are even less certain. Formal statistics on abuse and neglect are not available for most developing countries and the literature contains only references to specific case studies (Maroulis, 1979; Okeahialam, 1984). Nwako (1974) tallied 2,462 cases of accidental injury reported to a large hospital in Nigeria over a two-year period, of which 50 were judged to be examples of abuse. Prompted by a debate over definitions, more recent studies have attempted to place child abuse in non-Western societies in a wider anthropological context (Korbin, 1981).

The lack of any formal or legal requirement on reporting in many countries continues to hinder any viable international comparison of incidence rates. However, a very comprehensive international survey of infant and child mortality carried out by Christoffel et al. (1981), using WHO statistics, made a comparison of rates for 52 countries for definite inflicted injury (AE148) and possible inflicted injury (AE149). Details of some of their findings for 1972–1974, compared with similar data for 1980–1982 abstracted by the present author, are given in Tables 1A and 1B.

Care must be taken in interpreting these data, since they are likely to be subject to systematic bias in reporting. They do, however, suggest that abuse may be more prevalent in the industrialized countries than in the developing world. Also, they show an overall increase in the rates during the last decade in developing and the developed countries, with the increase being more marked for the Third World countries.

Some comments on the variations in estimates of incidence of abuse

Allusion was made earlier to the lack of any uniform definition of abuse and the resultant bias this has introduced to the establishment of reliable and valid incidence data. Even where investigators have restricted their attention to cases

Table 1A. Proportion of childhood deaths due to definite (AE148) and possible (AE149) inflicted injury, in developing and developed countries. Data for 1972–1974. (After Christoffel et al., 1981).

Category		AE148		AE149	
		Under 1 yr	1–4 yrs	Under 1 yr	1–4 yrs
Developing	(23)	0.04%	0.025%	0.08%	0.74%
Developed	(24)	0.17%	1.25%	0.05%	0.38%

Note: data under 1 year based on rate per 100 000 live births

which may be diagnosed more objectively under the classic rubric of 'battered baby syndrome' on the basis of frank physical injury, data relating to fundamental demographic characteristics (such as age, sex, socioeconomic status) are often lacking in subsequent analyses. Many researchers have adopted a restricted definition of abuse, which centres on infant cases — it still remains unclear whether the incidence of abuse diminishes with chronological age as a consequence of a reduction in the frequency of incidents or as a result of increased physical resilience in the putative victims.

Table 1B. Proportion of childhood deaths due to homicide (and injury purposely inflicted by other persons) and to other violence, in developed and developing countries. Date for 1980–1982 (WHO, 1984).

Category		HOMICIDE		OTHER VIOLENCE	
		Under 1 yr	1–4 yrs	Under 1 yr	1–4 yrs
Developing	(24)	0.08%	0.35%	0.22%	1.80%
Developed	(19)	0.24%	2.11%	0.11%	0.53%

Note: data under 1 year based on rate per 100 000 live births

It has long been recognized that incidence rates are distorted by both underreporting and misdiagnosis, although with increasing professional awareness this appears to be less of a problem than formerly. However, it remains a matter of concern that a significant number of cases are missed because the parents or guardians do not attend for treatment, or may use different hospitals or services on repeated occasions. Newberger and Hyde (1975) provide evidence of lack of coordination in reporting systems even where there is a legal requirement of notification, supported by sophisticated data-handling systems. In this respect, Gelles (1979) outlines six systems which are likely to be involved in identifying, labelling, treating and preventing child abuse: the medical system (public and private), the social-welfare system, the legal system (courts and police), the school/educational system, the neighbourhood system, and the family-kinship system.

The practical consequences of detection must, according to Gelles (1979), be assessed with respect to its likely error rate: in the case of false positives the 'accused' guardian or parent may be liable to stigmatization, whereas the false-negative instance could have disastrous consequences for the child — as has often happened in the United Kingdom, resulting in a number of official inquiries into the conduct and efficacy of welfare agencies. Light (1973) has suggested that screening programmes for abuse must first aim at a reduction of the false-negative rates, leaving false positives to be followed up later. This point will be discussed further in relation to prevention programmes.

In view of the wide variation in the estimates of abuse, both national and internationally, it is difficult to determine whether abuse is on the increase or waning. Even where reporting is legally required the data are liable to bias from procedure and practice. The usefulness of incidence rates as a basis for preventive and treatment programmes must be regarded with some doubt. Indeed, incidence and prevalence data illustrate forcefully the problem of generalizability of much research into child abuse.

SOME PREDICTIVE FACTORS IN CHILD ABUSE

A number of points should be borne in mind with regard to the voluminous literature on putative factors in child abuse. First, the overwhelming majority of studies are retrospective, and analyses of behaviour after the event risk confounding the behaviour with the explanation. Retrospective studies may often be based on biased samples — parents/guardians who have come under the scrutiny of the authorities as abusers, under whatever definition of abuse is current. Many subject samples are small, although aggregate samples will accrue from continuing research. Moreover, although more recent research has increasingly been based on control-group comparison, there is little agreement on what constitutes an appropriate control group for a child-abuse sample. Some studies have used control groups of non-abusing parents or guardians, others have used non-abused-children groups. Since abusive behaviour, in most Western societies, usually results in some involvement of the legal system, a more appropriate control group might be one recruited from those individuals who, like abusers, are caught up in this process.

In this section, some factors which may be of use in predicting which children, guardians or families may be at risk for abuse are outlined and discussed. Equally, some consideration is given to variables which have little or only restrictive value in explaining the aetiology of abuse.

The range of variables considered is not exhaustive, but is intended to illustrate the multifactorial nature of the problem. The approach will be to move from micro- to macro-levels of explanation: this corresponds to the three main levels of analysis which have evolved in child-abuse research in the last two decades and includes medical/intra-individual models, and sociopsychological and socio-cultural models (Gelles and Cornell, 1983). Finally an integration of the material will be proposed in consideration of the social ecological model of abuse.

Personality and psychopathological factors

The psychiatric approach to abuse, variously termed the psychopathological or psychodynamic model (Gelles, 1973; Sweet and Resick, 1979) can be character-ized as a relatively simple linear model in which societal factors play a minimal role, if any.

Early work in this area was based on the assumption of 'a general defect in character structure' (Spinetta and Rigler, 1972) although, as Wolfe (1985) points out, in the absence of hard evidence. The concept of character disorder was gradually replaced during the 1970s by reference to terms such as inadequacy, poor impulse-control and immaturity. Latterly, more attention has been paid to situational factors involving cognitive and emotional functioning and the interaction between stable personality traits and stressful life-events. Such studies, which are noteworthy in the use of control-group methodology, have in the main been unable to determine any significant group-differences in personality characteristics between abusing and non-abusing parents (Starr, 1982; Wright, 1976). However, some studies have indicated raised levels of somatic symptomatology and non-specific distress in abusive parents (Conger et al., 1979; Lahey et al., 1984).

Green et al. (1980) in a recent study attempted to distinguish between abusive, neglectful and control mothers. They drew subjects from a larger sample of 240 mothers and investigated them by means of a standardized clinical interview procedure — the Current and Past Psychopathology Scales (CAPPS) — in which all interviewing and rating was carried out blindly. They found no significant differences between the groups for the current evaluation, but they found group differences for three of the past scales, namely neurotic childhood, disorganiza-tion, and anger-excitability. Nevertheless, despite encouraging step-wise mul-tiple discriminant analysis classifications which did discriminate between the groups, Green et al. (1980) state that the degree of accuracy in classification (approximately 60%) does not justify the use of lengthy interview procedures and sophisticated judges for case identification. In a considered discussion of their own study they conclude that the attribution of maltreatment to the 'abuse-prone personality' (Gaines et al., 1978) is not warranted, and that the failure of abusers and neglectors to show significantly more frank psychopathology on scales that indicate more severe disturbance contradicts many reports in the clinical literature.

The typological approach to child abuse has maintained an important position in the scientific debate concerning aetiology. Certainly, the methodological basis of many early studies is open to question, where conclusions were based on restricted and, in some cases, highly selected groups, and often without reference to control groups. In later, more controlled studies the absence of frank psychopathology is matched by the frequency with which quasi-personality factors are observed — factors which are more related to diffuse psychosocial variables than to specific personality characteristics. In a review of psychiatric and personality research, which covered a period up to 1973, Parke and Collmer (1975) concluded that reservations ought to be made concerning the usefulness of the personality approach to child abuse. Evidence from studies in the intervening decade can only serve to reinforce rather than allay their original doubts.

Alcohol and drug abuse

Fetal injury consequent to the abuse of alcohol and drugs by pregnant mothers has been long suspected, and recent research on the 'fetal alcohol syndrome' has pointed out the long-term neuropsychological damage which may ensue. It has now become accepted by workers in the field that alcohol and drug misuse by pregnant mothers may be viewed as a 'special' form of child abuse. A significant review in this area is provided by Black and Mayer (1980).

Concern in this present paper will be for alcohol and drug misuse as mediating variables in the elicitation of physical abuse or neglect towards the young child.

Westermeyer and Bearman (1973) proposed that, because of the association between alcoholism and child abuse observed in many clinical case-studies, incidence rates for child abuse could be used as an indicator of the prevalence of alcoholism. Presumably, if a causal relationship does exist between the two variables, the reverse would also hold: regrettably, the question of definition within the field of alcoholism is as problematical as that for child abuse, where definitions range from clinically diagnosed alcoholism to 'problem' or 'excessive' drinking. The methodological difficulties inherent in this area are highlighted by Orme and Rimmer (1981), who also provide an extensive review of the literature.

Nevertheless, there have been a series of empirical studies which have investigated the role which alcohol abuse may play in potentiating violence towards the child. Some studies derive from alcoholism research where the primary interest was not in child abuse, but where retrospective accounts of childhood by the offspring of alcoholics include reference to physical abuse (Booz-Allen and Hamilton, 1974), or where high levels of intrafamilial violence are reported for parents undergoing treatment for alcoholism (Wilson and Orford, 1978).

One of the earliest studies on abuse and neglect (Young, 1964), based on case records, found that a high percentage of families (over 50%) included severe or chronic drinkers. More recent studies have found that alcohol abuse is implicated to varying degrees, ranging from a high of 69% of cases (Behling, 1979) to lows of 2–4% (Scott, 1973; Steele and Pollock, 1974). Several studies employ the concept of 'overflow abuse' (Delsordo, 1963) to encompass a complex of behaviours, including severe drinking, drug misuse and violence. A number of case studies indicate that alcohol abuse may be more prevalent amongst fathers than mothers in abusive families (Elmer, 1967; Johnson and Morse, 1968), but no empirical evidence has been presented in the literature.

There have been few attempts to address the role of alcohol or drug abuse within a theoretical framework of child abuse and neglect. A notable exception to this is recent work by Lesnik-Oberstein et al. (1982), whose 'aggression inhibition' model specifically posits substance misuse as a contributory factor in the disinhibition of violent behaviour in abusive parents.

The evidence for a link between child abuse and neglect and alcohol or drug abuse must still be regarded as one of association and not causation. There is evidently some scope for collaborative efforts between researchers in the two areas to provide more empirical evidence to support the observations of clinicians and other professional care-workers.

The special case of the 'special child'

It would be incautious to suggest that evidence concerning the role of the child in abuse has been consolidated into a comprehensive theory similar to those proposed to account for the role of the abusive parent. Nevertheless, increasing

51

attention has been paid to the possibility that the victim may be instrumental in some way in eliciting attack or neglect.

As Friedrich and Boroskin (1976) point out in a comprehensive review of the topic, the infant or young child, for a complex of reasons, may not be or provide the salubrious and benign stimulus which the parent may have been led to expect, or indeed, to demand.

They identified five main characteristics which may contribute to a child being viewed as 'special' or 'particular' in some way: these include prematurity or other perinatal complications, mental retardation, physical handicap or ill-health, individual differences which are possibly genetically determined, and parental perception of the child. This typology of the 'special' abused child differs radically from that often advanced for the abusive parent, in that these features can for the most part the objectively assessed as being present before the abuse incident occurred.

Several studies have found prematurity and other perinatal complications to be associated with abuse (Elmer and Gregg, 1967: Lynch and Roberts, 1977; Soumenkoff et al., 1982; Stern, 1973). The pre-term infant is often subject to a range of neonatal problems, such as colic, anoxia, viral or bacterial infection; developmental difficulties in visual and auditory responsiveness, increased muscle tension or sensitivity to pain and handling may be apparent in the first few days of life. Disturbance of sleep patterns has been observed frequently in premature infants (Dreyfus-Brisac, 1974). However, a recent retrospective study by Benedict et al. (1985) of 532 abused children showed that selected medical definitions of abnormal pregnancy, labour and delivery did not discriminate families at risk for maltreatment, although abusing mothers did have shorter birth intervals, less prenatal care and a history of previous stillbirths or repeated abortions.

The extent to which neonatal problems persist into early childhood or manifest themselves, perhaps as hyperactivity, later in development remains equivocal (Sameroff and Chandler, 1975): it is of note that some longitudinal studies indicate that social status factors may reduce or exacerbate the impact of perinatal trauma.

It is not inconceivable that some perinatal features could place an overwhelming burden on the ability of some parents to give children care. The possible interaction of these infant characteristics and the occurrence of post-partum depression has received some attention (Asch and Rubin, 1974; Gray et al., 1979). A prospective study of 150 mothers (Gray et al., 1979) assigned to high-and low-risk groups on the basis of perinatal and questionnaire data has shown that post-partum depression was reported for a significantly higher percentage of the high-risk mothers (74%) than for the low-risk group (44%). Furthermore, 46% of the high-risk mothers described the first few days at home with the new infant as a negative experience, while only 8% of the low-risk mothers did so. There appear to be few systematic studies of child abuse related to menstruation (Dalton, 1975).

Separation of the mother and child, normally as a consequence of abnormal delivery or prematurity, has also been considered in relation to child abuse in terms of both emotional bonding (Ounsted et al., 1974) and subsequent material behaviour. A follow-up study of 146 mothers of low-birth-weight babies (Fanaroff et al., 1972) warrants consideration: over a two-week period mothers who visited their child less than three times were noted. Out of 11 subsequent abuse and neglect cases in this series, nine were mothers who had been infrequent visitors.

Although a number of studies have reported an increased frequency of mental retardation among abused children (Sandgrund et al., 1974) there is a very real possibility that congenital dysfunction is confounded with the effects of sustained abuse over time. However, congenital physical abnormalities have been associated with the abused child: Lynch (1975) reported a high incidence of severe cleft palate and hare-lip. There is also some evidence (Lynch, 1975) that serious or recurrent illness (pneumonia, bronchitis, non-specific convulsions) is more frequent in abused children compared with their sibling controls — it remains a possibility, however, as Howells (1975) suggested, that these illnesses are a secondary cause of abuse and may have stemmed from neglect. The point at issue, then, is whether some abused children are different in some characteristic way from their non-abused peers and siblings, or whether a parent judges them as being different. The evidence from Lynch (1975), who used sibling controls, suggests real differences in terms of physical illness during the first year of life. Morse et al. (1970) found in 25 cases that six children were thought by the parents to be 'bad', 'selfish', 'spoiled rotten' and defiant in comparison with their siblings. Parental expectations about child development must be considered as a factor in child abuse. De Lissavoy (1973) found unrealistic expectations to be common (especially in fathers) including beliefs that a baby would be able to sit alone at 12 weeks, take the first step alone at 40 weeks, and perhaps more important in this context, be able to recognize wrongdoing at 52 wccks. The attribution of deliberate intent on the child's behalf was frequent.

It is evident that the role the child may play, either actively or by default, in eliciting abuse must continue to be considered in research on aetiology. Such research on the 'special' child at risk may contribute to our knowledge of why in multi-member families one child often seems to fulfil the role of scapegoat, the other children remaining unscathed (Gil, 1970: Lynch, 1975). It is important to note that no single causal factor has emerged from this area of research, and that terms such as 'bonding failure' or 'attachment' should be applied cautiously since they often imply a unicausal process. Emphasis must be placed on the interactive and multidimensional aspects of child-rearing where a dynamic relationship exists between the child and parents/guardians from the very earliest point of development.

Social interaction analyses

A large body of research has been directed to the microanalysis of interactions between guardians and children in abusive and non-abusive families. Two main currents underlie much of this research: the first derives from social learning theorists (Bandura, 1977: Stein and Friedrich, 1975) and provides the theoretical base for modelling or generational theories of abuse. The second approach directs attention to factors which are viewed as predisposing but which are not themselves sufficient for abuse to take place (Vasta, 1982), such as a stress-loaded environment or inappropriate child-rearing practices and interpersonal behaviours.

Empirical evidence for the thesis that abuse is generational is provided from several studies of abusing parents which show that the perpetrators were themselves abused as children (Green et al., 1974; Hyman, 1978; Jameson and Schellenbach, 1977). Hyman's (1978) study of social work schedules from 85 cases known to the National Society for the Prevention of Cruelty to Children (NSPCC) found that 31% of the mothers reported abuse in their own childhood.

Support for atypical levels of family violence in abusive families was also evidenced in this study, where 41% of the mothers reported violence against them by their partner. Jameson and Schellenbach (1977) carried out separate analyses for male (n=46) and female (n=36) abusers: a significant difference in childhood history of abuse was found for females (66%) but not for the males (46%). In contrast, Kadushin and Martin (1981) found less support for the intergenerational theory in their study of 66 abuse cases, where only 25% of the parents reported mistreatment as children.

The social psychological model of abuse, outlined by Gelles (1973), places some importance on situational stress as a primary factor in abusive behaviour. Conger et al. (1979) used indices of life-changes as an indicator of social stress and suggested that life-changes in interaction with a punitive family history may result in abusive acts on the part of the parent. Their sample was small (n=20) but it was found that abusive parents were more likely to have experienced both a series of rapid life-changes and a history of punitive rearing in their own childhood. Personal injury or illness contributed most to the life-event scores, as well as their having higher ill-health scores on the Cornell Medical Index. However, Conger et al. (1979) postulate that, while life crises, ill-health and punitive history may precipitate abuse, the immediate situation may provide "the grist which determines whether a parent will physically injure the child" (p. 77).

One aspect of the pathway to abuse which is receiving more attention is that of the 'immediate situation' — case histories of abusive behaviour are replete with accounts of child behaviour which parents viewed as major transgressions and to which they reacted accordingly. Kadushin and Martin (1981) tabulate the immediate precursors of abuse in their series of 66 cases, where the largest single category (accounting for 21% of abusive incidents) was aggressive behaviour by the child, either verbal or physical.

This class of behaviour seems to accord well with what Frude (1978) has termed "instrumental aggression" where the parent commits an aggressive act in anticipation of positive pay-offs (for example, a cessation of 'deliberate' crying). An unrealistic demand may obviate a viable or realistic response by the child and set the stage for conflict when the parent's power is effectively challenged, either intentionally or unintentionally. It is possible to envisage such an incident where instrumental aggression and anger aggression could rapidly escalate and interact to a point where only very strong inhibitory factors would reduce the likelihood of physical assault. Mechanisms of inhibition in such situations are poorly understood: Frude (1978) has suggested that inhibitions may be progressively lowered over time as maltreatment continues without serious consequences. Smith and Hanson (1975) have also pointed to the abusive parent's inconsistency towards the child, and the inconsistent use of instrumental and anger aggression could perhaps explain why some older abused children display 'frozen watchfulness' (Ounstead et al., 1974) as a strategy for coping with unpredictable behaviour by the parent.

Demographic and societal factors

The sociological approach to child abuse is founded on the assumption that societal variables are paramount as primary determinants of child abuse and neglect. Essentially, the research has centred on two main propositions: that socioeconomic status, or, more properly, social-class structure, acts as a determinant of abuse, and that the status of violence as legitimate behaviour co-varies with the likelihood of abuse in children. Additionally, much sociological research has drawn on demographic data to expand the characterization of the abusive family and its members.

Comprehensive reviews of the demographic data have been given by Parke and Collmer (1975) and Sweet and Resick (1979). Only brief mention of some salient details will be made here.

Characteristically, the abused child is quite young, most notified cases being under two years of age (Baldwin and Oliver, 1975; Smith and Deasy, 1977); however, Morgan (1978) draws attention to adolescent cases and suggests that as many as 30% of the total population of abused children may be older than 12 years. In younger age groups of abused children there appears to be some evidence that the male child is more at risk, although only marginally so. In the study by Baldwin and Oliver (1975) both retrospective and prospective samples were employed — boys outnumbered girls in the retrospective series (1.4:1.0) but there were more abused females in the prospective sample (1.0:1.7). Creighton (1979) found a boy:girl ratio of 5:4 for cases recorded by the NSPCC in the United Kingdom. Benedict et al. (1985) in a study of perinatal risk factors report that 59% of their sample of mothers with children under four years of age consisted of boys.

Most studies in the United Kingdom (Creighton, 1979; Hyman, 1978) suggest that the abusive mother is younger (early twenties) than the national average for mothers with a dependent child under five years of age. Abusive fathers tend to be somewhat older. Bolton et al. (1980) have suggested that the child of an adolescent mother may be at higher risk, but Kinard and Klerman (1980) conclude that the association between teenage pregnancy and child abuse may be confounded in each case with social class.

Similarly, there is some evidence that mothers are more likely to be involved in abusive acts than fathers. Benedict et al. (1985) report that in 38.7% of the cases the mother was identified as the abuser compared with 18.4% cases involving the father. However, when all males are taken into account (including stepfathers and boy-friends) the male involvement rises to 31%. Cases involving both parents accounted for only 2.5%. In contrast, Creighton (1979) found that mothers or mother substitutes were suspected in 44% of cases compared with 46.5% of cases involving fathers or father substitutes.

Some studies relating to family structure (Baldwin and Oliver, 1975; Creighton, 1979) suggest that the abused child is more likely to come from a large family. Several reports indicate a higher degree of mobility in abusive families: Hyman (1978) found that one third of abusive families had moved twice or more in the preceding three years, and Creighton (1979) found that only 8% of the abusive families had lived in one place for over five years, compared with 70% for manual workers in general. Instability in family structure has also been noted (Baldwin and Oliver, 1975), with higher rates of divorce, separation and cohabitation. Creighton (1979) found that only 52% of the children were living with both biological parents at the time of the incident, 22% with their mother and a father substitute, and 20% with a single parent. In the Benedict et al. (1985) study from the Baltimore district of Maryland over 40% of the cases were observed in single-parent families, compared with 25.2% where both parents were present. Sills et al. (1977) recorded higher levels of illegitimacy in a sample of Liverpool cases, and Hyman (1978) reports an illegitimacy rate in abusive families of four times the national UK average (39% versus 9%).

Unemployment has been advanced as a potential social stressor in child abuse (Parke and Collmer, 1975). However, Baldwin and Oliver (1975) stated that they found it difficult to evaluate the occupational histories of fathers or father substitutes in their study, as the sample was marked by frequent job changes and periods of unemployment. Hyman (1978) found that, where the male was in employment, hours worked were often high on average (53 hours) compared with the national average (45.5 hours). Unemployment has been suggested as a major determinant of intra-family violence (Steinmetz and Straus, 1974) since it often involves a perceived loss of status which may be compensated for by attempts to increase authority in the home. However, it may be that unemployment results in the father coming into more frequent contact with children in the home and thereby the opportunity for conflict situations to arise may be increased. Gelles (1979) has warned of the temptation to make a simple comparison between unemployment rates and abuse rates, which may show a simultaneous increase, since this does not allow for any conclusions about individual behaviour and abuse but commits the ecological fallacy.

The most comprehensive treatment of socioeconomic status and abuse, drawing largely on evidence from the U.S.A., is provided by Pelton's (1978) critique of the 'myth of classlessness'. Utilizing survey data, Pelton found that only 3% of the sample had incomes over US$10 000 compared with about one third of the national population. The American Humane Association's (1978) report on over 12 000 cases of abuse indicated that over half of the families had a yearly income below 5 000 dollars.

However, Gil (1975) identified poverty as only one of several 'triggering contexts', in his sociocultural model of child abuse. This formulation is the most socially oriented of all the various models which have been advanced to account for child abuse and distinguishes five levels of causation. At the interpersonal level, the theory accepts a causal contribution from 'intrapsychic conflicts and various forms of psychopathology' (p. 13), but Gil stresses that such disturbances are deeply rooted in, and constantly interact with, forces in the social environment of the disturbed individual (p. 14). A second causal dimension is the trigger context of social stressors which includes overcrowding, abnormal family structure, economic stringency and work alienation. A third causal dimension centres on the social acceptance of force as a legitimate way of achieving a goal, especially within power structures already established in a given society, such as the male-female and parent-child relationships. Closely allied to this level of causation is the fourth, which relates to the social construction of childhood in a given society.

The most fundamental and powerful causal level for Gil, however, is a society's basic 'social philosophy, its dominant value premises, its concept of humans; the nature of its social, economic and political institutions . . .' (p. 9).

The sociological approach to child abuse has developed along two main dimensions. The first has attempted empirically to determine the relationship between various socio-demographic factors and abuse, with special attention to the role of poverty and social deprivation. The second approach remains to a large extent theoretical and postulates that the social philosophy of a given society is the prime determinant of abuse. In this respect, it would be apposite to test the assumption by reference to more cross-cultural studies.

In many ways the debate concerning social factors and abuse parallels that in the psychiatric literature concerning the relationship between psychopathology and social class. It may be well to heed the advice of Dohrenwend and Dohrenwend (1974), who stated that the basic issues concerning the role of social factors (in psychopathology) would not be settled until attention was moved away from cross-sectional surveys to quasi-experimental designs, which exploit the contrasts provided by concurrent social processes and allow for the testing of specific alternative hypotheses.

The ecology of child abuse

The ecological framework has been proposed by Belsky (1980) as a way of integrating the ostensibly divergent and discrepant research findings on abuse and neglect. It emphasizes the analysis of the interaction between the child and the environment or contexts in which the child lives.

The environment is conceived as an arrangement of interacting systems, nested within each other — the micro-system, the exo-system and the macro-system. The micro-system represents the family setting in which abuse takes place. The exo-system encompasses the concurrent social structure, which might include the neighbourhood, the employment situation, etc. The macro-system incorporates the sociocultural beliefs and values which may engender or promote the occurrence of abuse.

Initially, it may appear that this model of abuse and neglect differs little from those proposed by sociological analyses. There is, however, no presumption that any one level is more determinant than another, since the ecological model assumes a dynamic of interdependent and interacting systems. More important, the model allows a distinction between the necessary and the sufficient conditions for abuse to take place. Given a sufficient condition, for example a parent's reliance on, and use of, corporal punishment, abuse is less likely to occur in the absence of a necessary condition such as family isolation from potent support systems, for, as Garbarino (1977) points out, 'Child abuse feeds on privacy'.

Belsky (1980) presents an attempt to integrate the diversity of findings on abuse under the ecological model: for example, studies relating to unemployment and social isolation, both implicated in abuse, are subsumed at the exo-system level but may interact at both the micro-system level, where personality factors may underlie interpersonal isolation, and the macro-system level through a society's endorsement of the nuclear family.

Although it is unlikely that we have enough control over real-life situations to be able to establish directionality of effect in an experimental fashion (Baumrind, 1980), major shifts in a given society's social philosophy, as in the child-oriented legislation promulgated in Sweden, provide the setting for what Bronfenbrenner (1977) has termed the 'ecological experiment'. In this vein, Garbarino (1977) set out a schema for conducting and evaluating future research in abuse and neglect. His main concern is to reorient research away from the study of individual and family characteristics towards an analysis of geopolitical units (e.g., counties within states), communities and neighbourhoods (whether defined naturally or phenomenologically), and families as interacting systems in their own right.

Efforts to achieve a comprehensive model of child abuse are undoubtedly seen at their most ambitious in the contributions of human ecologists. The integrative nature of the model brings together most coherently the large corpus of findings which have accumulated from disparate theoretical (and atheoretical) approaches to the problem. While the ecological theory gives equal consideration to each of the putative systems which may underpin or sustain abuse and neglect, in practice it has focused mainly on the family micro-system and the community exo-system levels. This has been the case especially with regard to intervention and prevention programmes (Gray et al., 1977; Olds, 1978).

The extent to which the ecological perspective is successful in promoting a more integrated approach to research into child abuse and in formulating specific preventive measures remains to be demonstrated: however, Ziegert's (1983) ecological analysis of the Swedish legislation on corporal punishment demonstrates the usefulness of this kind of theoretical analysis to real-life conditions.

The ecological model offers more than simply the opportunity to systematize what is already known — it also suggests a new perspective in which maltreatment can be seen as a developmental issue (at both the micro- and the macro-level). Here, the model returns a measure of specificity to an area which is always in danger of becoming overgeneralized — for example, 'they must be mad' or 'it's all the fault of unemployment' — since it proposes a nested set of structures and processes. A dysfunction such as child abuse can be located within a given level and the reciprocating links between levels can be elucidated.

Sweet and Resick (1979) concluded their review of child abuse with the statement that 'the causal relations [which] sociological theories imply . . . are quite impossible to change' (p. 55). They cite specifically both poverty and violence. One major proposition of the ecological approach confronts this pessimism, since it calls for 'experiments' which involve the restructuring of prevailing systems, such as changes in family law and children's rights. The extent to which the ecologically driven intervention and prevention studies address these issues will be the ultimate test of the model's validity and claim to social relevance.

CONSEQUENCES OF ABUSE

This section deals with some studies which have considered the prognosis for a child who has suffered abuse and neglect.

It may be apposite, however, at this point to reflect for a moment on the immediate consequences for the victims of abuse and neglect, before turning to more subtle long-term effects. The primary effects of abuse are temporary or permanent bodily injuries, which may occur singly or in combination and which differ in degree of severity. Some children may present with a history of abuse which has been inflicted over a period of time. Cooper (1978) lists some of the following: bruises, lacerations, wheals, burns and scalds, fractures and joint injury, abdominal and chest injuries, and head injuries including haematomas and ocular damage. The list is not exhaustive — to it could be added less specific damage as a result of poisoning or attempted drowning and suffocation.

Consequences of neglect range from the specific physical conditions seen in deprivational dwarfism to chronic or acute malnutrition and hypothermia. Again, this is not a complete list, but one which illustrates the diversity seen in the immediate after-effects of neglect. Some of the outcomes, both physical and psychosocial, are listed below: it should be noted that many of the sequelæ are interdependent but may follow different temporal sequences.

Some sequelæ of non-accidental injury

Physical—Ocular damage; aural damage; bone deformity; scars; paraplegia; growth dysfunction; neurological dysfunction; developmental retardation.

Psychosocial—Developmental retardation; minimal brain dysfunction; cognitive/intellectual dysfunction; hyperactivity/hypoactivity; emotional/affective disturbance; aggressiveness; delinquency; substance abuse.

Again, as with other research areas in abuse, a note of caution must be raised concerning some of the methodological weaknesses to which studies are prone — small samples, only restricted follow-up, and inappropriate assessment methods. Nevertheless, there is some evidence which hints at significant long-term effects on physical, cognitive and social development in abused children. Toro (1982) has provided a critical review of studies to which the interested reader might refer.

Among the first to carry out studies on the sequelæ of abuse and neglect was Elmer (1967), using a retrospective follow-up of 22 severe cases of abuse. The results of this study showed that almost a third of the children presented the 'failure to thrive syndrome', just over half had IQ scores below 80, and half had speech or language problems. Other negative features in these children included angry outbursts and behaviour problems at school.

In a later study by Martin et al. (1974), which included a follow-up neurological examination, some 43% of the cases, without a history of previous head trauma, showed some neurological dysfunction. Buchanan and Oliver (1977) surveyed 140 children under 16 years of age in two subnormality hospitals and concluded that in 11% of the cases the handicap could have been the result of abuse. Gross and persistent central nervous system dysfunction was found in five of 16 abused children and another four were borderline mental retardates with severe behaviour problems — one child in this latter group was known to have suffered at least 10 episodes of head injury before the age of five. Neglect was considered to be a contributory factor to borderline retardation for 12% of the sample, and Buchanan and Oliver (1977) stress the need for recognition of the combined effects of abuse and neglect, especially for those children who may already be at high risk as a result of prenatal and perinatal insult.

Results comparable to those quoted above have been found in a series of studies which have dealt with cognitive and emotional functioning in abused children: Kline (1977) studied 137 cases and found 27% of the sample were in special classes for the educationally subnormal, learning disabled or emotionally disturbed, and that 70% of these children were below their grade for mathematics and reading. Martin and Beezley (1977) reported that over half their follow-up sample exhibited school learning problems and behaviour which led to their rejection by teachers and peers.

A study of teachers' attitudes to abused children and their siblings (Roberts et al., 1976) showed that many are judged hostile and suffer social isolation, possibly as a consequence of higher levels of aggression. Support for this comes from George and Main (1979), who observed that by 13 to 35 months of age a sample of abused children was displaying more aggression to guardians and peers in a day-care setting than was a matched control group.

A possible link between childhood abuse and subsequent anti-social behaviour, such as adolescent delinquency and substance abuse, has been proposed by a number of authors. Lewis et al. (1979) found that 75% of their sample of delinquent youths had themselves been abused. Cohen and Densen-Gerber (1982) investigated 177 patients undergoing treatment for alcohol and drug abuse, of whom 84% reported a history of abuse during childhood. These findings lend support to the inter-generational hypotheses of abusive behaviour.

Despite the many methodological difficulties which follow-up studies encounter, there is some evidence that child abuse is detrimental to a range of developmental processes. Studies of frank subnormality or mental retardation — for example, that of Eppler and Brown (1977) in Alaska attributed some 15% of cases to abuse and neglect — indicate a primary cause to be physical abuse. However, other studies suggest that the long-term effects of abuse may be non-specific and diffuse in many of the children. There is some evidence to suggest that differences in functioning may be heavily influenced by situational factors, either in the home or in given test situations. Baron et al. (1970), for example, found that neurological dysfunction quickly remitted when children were admitted to hospital.

More recently, Elmer (1977), in a long-term prospective study of abused children and non-abused accident controls, has found with repeated follow-ups that the initial differences between the groups as regards health and emotional lability decrease — although both groups showed considerable deficits overall, which Elmer concluded were due rather to low socioeconomic status and associated social stresses than to abuse *per se.*

While there is evidence of some important sequelæ to childhood abuse, caution must be exercised as regards cause and effect and the influence of confounding variables such as socioeconomic status and other related factors. There is a need for more longitudinal assessment in follow-up studies, as in Elmer (1977), rather than reliance on single-point investigations: if the latter are used they should include repeated measures as a minimum requirement. A combination of cross-sectional and sequential strategies would be the optimal research path in this area.

PREVENTION OF CHILD ABUSE

In their review of primary prevention in the mental health field, Kessler and Albee (1975) emphasized that the explanatory models used to account for disorder have profound implications for prevention strategies. The same is true of preventive measures in child abuse, where programmes could be instituted at the various levels of analysis outlined previously — the level of the individual, family or society. Further, as Helfer (1982) points out, preventive programmes may be aimed at either reduction or minimization of abuse *per se,* or at an enhancement of positive interaction between the parties involved.

Programmes for prevention of child abuse may be concerned with primary, secondary or tertiary prevention. The primary approach is aimed at preventing abuse and neglect from ever occurring, at the level of either the individual or the social group. Secondary prevention is aimed at those judged to be at some higher risk for abuse, and tertiary programmes would be concerned principally with the prevention of subsequent abuse in notified cases.

Our concern here will be to outline briefly some of the approaches at the primary and secondary levels. Preventive programmes, either operational or proposed, may be classified into a number of different categories. Helfer (1982) provides an extensive review of research in this area and may be consulted for additional details. Some possible preventive models are outlined below:

a) Child treatment and education programmes: these are aimed at the abused child or the child at risk, and include group therapy, play therapy, developmental enhancement procedures and such like. Programmes may be directed at the individual child, or may be organized on a wider basis to encompass special facilities, such as day-care centres, for children at risk. Programmes akin to Head Start and Upstart might also be considered in this category.

b) Perinatal and postnatal programmes: this approach draws heavily on research which indicates that early parent/baby bonding may be a crucial variable in predisposing individuals to abuse, and aims at an enhancement of positive interaction.

c) Multidisciplinary SCAN teams: drawing on the services of nurses, health visitors, paediatricians, social workers, police and other community workers may be advantageous not only in after-the-event care but also in preventing further or subsequent abuse by intervention.

d) Public education programmes: the educational system provides the opportunity for specific teaching programmes on child-care and rearing as well as specialist courses in the subject of abuse and neglect.

e) Socio-political programmes: essentially proposed for enactment at both national and international levels, these programmes call for significant changes in societal frameworks to minimize the acceptance and likelihood of abuse and neglect. A number of countries, for example Sweden (1979) and Denmark (1985), have enacted legislation which prohibits the use of physical punishment by guardians.

It may be useful to illustrate briefly one programme which Helfer (1982) quotes as being the classic study in preventive methodology. Gray et al. (1979) identified groups of high- and low-risk parents on the basis of perinatal data, nursery observation and parent interviews. They randomly assigned 50 high-risk mothers to an intervention group, a further 50 to a non-intervention group, matched with 50 low-risk control mothers. Intervention took the form of comprehensive health care and health visiting over a two-year follow-up period.

Amongst other outcomes, some 10% of the non-intervention group were admitted to hospital for serious injury (including fractured femur, subdural haematoma, third-degree burns), while neither of the other two groups needed treatment for similar injuries. Gray et al. (1979) conclude from the results of this study that the relatively modest intervention procedures seem to have prevented severe injury from taking place in the intervention high-risk group.

A number of studies have been carried out on attempts to screen for risk, using a variety of instruments (including interviews, questionnaires on parental practices, and observation) with selected samples of parents. Researchers then often proposed an extension of these procedures — especially when relatively high specificity and sensitivity values are obtained — to more representative samples of the population (Disbrow et al., 1977). However, as Gaines et al. (1978) and Light (1973) have indicated, there are considerable problems inherent in mass screening. For example, assuming an incidence rate of 1% for abuse, screening 100 000 families with the Disbrow et al. (1977) test-battery, which successfully classified over 86% of abusing parents, would result in 850 children being correctly identified as potentially abused, 150 potential cases being missed, and 10 890 children being classified as false positives. Starr (1979) made a similar calculation for his own screening instrument and questioned whether any present social service network could deal effectively with such an outcome.

Educational programmes represent the broadest attempt at prevention. However, there is as yet little information on how effective they are. Many projects have involved voluntary participation, and the possibility remains that they are being addressed to a self-selecting group who already possess, or are influenced differentially by, other (undetermined) factors that protect against abuse. There is no agreement on whether there is an optimal period for delivering such programmes, and almost nothing is known about their reliability or validity over long periods.

Kellmer-Pringle (1980) recently suggested that, although basic to the prevention of abuse, educational approaches must be viewed in the long term, and that a more immediate strategy founded on a right to an independent and legally recognized advocate to represent the interests of the child may be more advantageous. There is little doubt that such an 'ombudsman' could play a vital role in coordinating care and protection services for children at risk, who all too often, through a linking of misinformation, failure of communication, inter-service jealousy, and even frank disavowal of circumstances on occasion, become further confirmed cases of abuse and neglect in some central registry.

CONCLUSION AND DISCUSSION

It is apparent that significant methodological difficulties militate against definitive conclusions being drawn about the aetiology of abuse and neglect from many studies carried out during the last decade or so. Leventhal (1982) has provided a comprehensive review of this area and proposed a series of standards which should be aimed at in subsequent research. These include concern for definition of abusive behaviour and outcomes, employment of specific control groups, and delineation of clear temporal sequencing between risk factors and abuse.

The question of incidence is intractably bound up with the problem of definition, and valid international comparisons are to be made unless there is an internationally agreed definition (even if limited in its scope). It would be useful to have such a category of abuse and neglect included in national statistical reporting. Almost all studies of epidemiology and of aetiology are based on research from the developed countries, but there is evidence in the literature that this situation is changing (Korbin, 1981; Loening, 1981). In this respect, it would seem a prerequisite for validity and reliability that anthropological expertise be more actively sought and encouraged. Garbarino and Ebata (1983) have recently drawn particular attention to the impact that rapid social and technological change may have on traditional family structures and processes, and they call for urgent research in this area. It is of interest that these authors also allow a role for sociobiological factors (in terms of parental investment and kin selection) within a broader ecological model than that formulated previously by Garbarino (1977).

Theoretical approaches to child abuse and neglect have centred primarily on rather specific linear models, for example the 'psychopathological' and 'special child' theories. Their limitations have been alluded to previously. It is encouraging that more recently there has been a move towards the multivariate model, although this is often characterized by a degree of *ad hoc* modification as and when each new piece of evidence, either supportive or contradictory, has arisen. This might be taken to exemplify Kuhn's (1962) description of a 'paradigm-in-crisis'. An emergent and dominant paradigm can be identified in the ecological model of abuse and neglect (Belsky, 1980; Garbarino, 1977): this offers a dynamic framework which emphasizes the relationships between the individual child, parents or guardians, family and society.

It is unlikely that models founded on a concept of linear causation, however multivariate, will be able to accommodate in a satisfactory manner the changes in interpersonal behaviour that ensue from rapid and major flux in social systems, such as those in the traditional role of women as primary guardians, or urbanization and industrialization in a Third World society.

Studies of the outcomes of abuse and neglect have suggested that the consequences may be both real and severe, ranging from specific mental retardation in individuals to intergenerational transmission of the behaviours associated with abuse both within and between family units. However, many follow-up studies are subject to methodological difficulties of 'experimental mortality', and of temporal sequencing of cause and effect. Sustained and systematic longitudinal research is required.

The generalizability of many predictive studies is uncertain: cross-validation of findings remains the exception. Where attempts have been made to utilise and integrate current research findings as part of a preventive strategy, the process appears to be most effective at the level of both the specific and the general social support system. Increased social and paramedical support directed towards the family during the perinatal development of the child appears to be beneficial. A further source of prevention lies in the provision of specific educational programmes which foster realistic expectations of parenthood and improved child-rearing practices.

It is almost 25 years since Kempe and his colleagues published their seminal article on the 'battered child syndrome' (Kempe et al., 1962). What began as a speciality of paediatrics has become since then a semi-autonomous discipline, with its own 'house' journal and international society. Whereas 20 years ago the interested observer could turn to two or three, medically oriented, journals, the choice today runs to perhaps ten times that number, with a much broader orientation. This spread reflects the extent to which child abuse has rapidly become demedicalized in both theory and practice.

One consequence of this development has been a plethora of models and theories of abuse, drawing on a diversity of constructs ranging from learning theory to social deviancy. What began as an attempt to construct a systematic explanation of abuse has begun to show signs of becoming a series of somewhat disjointed and fragmented propositions. The comprehensive model based on the ecological approach (Belsky, 1980) offers an opportunity for future studies of abuse to progress, where each niche in the framework represents a valid area of interest, in relation both to basic research and to prevention and treatment programmes. This model is not an easy one: it is quite difficult to develop statistical methods for mapping reciprocities between its components and levels. At a practical level, it demands a considerable amount of time and sustained motivation, and needs multidisciplinary involvement.

Finally, this model is based on a specific concept of child abuse and neglect as a sociopolitical issue. One of its propositions is that understanding of a process can best be advanced by "experiments involving the innovative restructuring of prevailing ecological systems in ways that depart from existing institutional ideologies and structures" (Bronfenbrenner, 1977, p. 528). One ecological option which is open to every society is to carry out such an experiment by changing its present laws and statutes when these do not actively promote the child's best interests. Very few have done so.

References

American Humane Association, (1978) *National Analysis of Official Child Neglect and Abuse Reporting.* AHA, Denver.

Asch, S.S. & Rubin, L.J. (1974) Postpartum reactions: some unrecognised variations. *American Journal of Psychiatry, 131* (8): 870–4.

Baldwin, J.A. & Oliver, J.E. (1975) Epidemiology and family characteristics of severely-abused children. *British Journal of Preventive and Social Medicine, 29 (4): 205–21.*

Bandura, A. (1977) *Social Learning Theory.* Prentice-Hall, New York.

Baron, M.A. *et al.* (1970) Neurologic manifestations of the battered child syndrome. *Pediatrics, 45* (6): 1003–07.

Baumrind, D. (1980) New directions in socialization research. *American Psychologist, 35* (7): 639–52.

Behling, D.W. (1979) Alcohol abuse as encountered in 51 instances of reported child abuse. *Clinical Pediatrics, 18*: 90–91.

Belsky, J. (1980) Child maltreatment. *American Psychologist, 35* (7): 652–65.

Benedict, M.I. *et al.* (1985) Maternal perinatal risk factors and child abuse. *Child Abuse and Neglect, 9*: 217–24.

Black, R. & Mayer, J. (1980) Parents with special problems: alcoholism and opiate addiction. In: Kempe, C.H. & Helfer, R.E. (eds.). *The Battered Child.* University of Chicago Press, Chicago.

Bolton, F.G. *et al.* (1980) Child maltreatment risk among adolescent mothers: a study of reported cases. *American Journal of Orthopsychiatry, 50* (3): 489–504.

Booz-Allen & Hamilton Inc. (1974) An assessment of the needs of and resources for children of alcoholic parents. National Technical Information Service, Springfield.

Brodie, T. (1982) Israel's battered children. *Newsview, 111:* 16–17.

Bronfenbrenner, U. (1977) Toward an experimental ecology of human development. *American Psychologist, 32* (6): 513–31.

Buchanan, A. & Oliver, J.E. (1977) Abuse and neglect as a cause of mental retardation: a study of 140 children admitted to mental subnormality hospitals in Wiltshire. *British Journal of Psychiatry, 131:* 458–67.

Christoffel, K.K. *et al.* (1981) Epidemiology of fatal child abuse: international mortality data. *Journal of Chronic Diseases, 34:* 57–64.

Cohen, F.S. & Denson-Gerber, J. (1982) A study of the relationship between child abuse and drug addiction in 178 patients: preliminary results. *Child Abuse and Neglect, 6:* 383–87.

Conger, R.D. *et al.* (1979) Child abuse related to life change and perceptions of illness: some preliminary findings. *Family Coordinator. 28:* 73–78.

Cooper, C. (1978) Symptoms, signs and diagnosis of physical abuse. In: Carver, V. (ed.), *Child Abuse.* Open University Press, Milton Keynes.

Creighton, S.J. (1979) An epidemiological study of child abuse. *Child Abuse and Neglect, 3:* 601–05.

Dalton, K. (1975) Paramenstrual body battering. *British Medical Journal, 2* (5965): 279.

DeFrancis, V. (1963) *Child Abuse — Preview of a Nationwide Survey.* AHA, Denver.

De Lissavoy, V. (1973) Child care by adolescent parents. *Children Today, 2:* 22–25.

Delsordo, J.D. (1963) Protective casework for abused children. *Children, 10:* 213–18.

Disbrow, M.A. *et al.* (1977) Measuring components of parents' potential for child abuse and neglect. *Child Abuse and Neglect. 1:* 279–96.

Dohrenwend, B.P. & Dohrenwend, B.S. (1974) Social and cultural influences on psychopathology. *Annual Review of Psychology, 25:* 417–52.

Dreyfus-Brisac, C. (1974) Ontogenesis of sleep in human prematures after 32 weeks of conceptual age. *Developmental Psychobiology, 3:* 91–121.

Dubanoski, R.A. & Snyder, K. (1980) Patterns of child abuse in Japanese- and Samoan-Americans. *Child Abuse and Neglect, 4:* 217–25.

Elmer, E. (1967) *Children in Jeopardy.* University of Pittsburgh Press, Pittsburgh.

Elmer, E. (1974) Hazards in determining child abuse. In Leavitt, J.E. (ed.), *The Battered Child.* General Learning Press, New Jersey.

Elmer, E. (1977) *Fragile Familes, Troubled Children: The Aftermath of Infant Trauma.* University of Pittsburgh Press, Pittsburgh.

Elmer, E. & Gregg, G.S. (1967) Developmental characteristics of abused children. *Pediatrics, 40* (4): 596–602.

Eppler, M. & Brown. G. (1977) Child abuse and neglect: preventable causes of mental retardation. *Child Abuse and Neglect, 1:* 309–13.

Fanaroff, A., Kennell, J.H. & Klaus, M.H. (1972) Follow-up of low weight infants — the predictive value of maternal visiting practices. *Pediatrics, 49* (2): 287–90.

Fergusson, D.M., Fleming, J. & O'Neill, D.P. (1972) *Child Abuse in New Zealand: Report on a Nationwide Survey of the Physical Ill-treatment of Children.* Shearer, Wellington.

Field, T. (1983) Child abuse in monkeys and humans: a comparative perspective. In: Reite, M. & Caine, N.G. (eds), *Child Abuse: The Nonhuman Primate Data.* Liss, New York.

Friedrich, W.N. & Boroskin, J.A. (1976) The role of the child in abuse: a review of the literature. *American Journal of Orthopsychiatry, 46* (4): 580–90.

Frude, N. (1978) *The aggression incident: a perspective for understanding abuse.* Paper presented at the Second International Congress on Child Abuse and Neglect, London.

Gaines, R. *et al,* (1978) Etiological factors in child maltreatment: a multivariate study of abusing, neglecting and normal mothers. *Journal of Abnormal Psychology. 87* (5): 531–40.

Garbarino, J. (1977) The human ecology of child maltreatment. *Journal of Marriage and the Family, 39:* 721–35.

Garbarino, J. & Ebata, A. (1983) The significance of ethnic and cultural differences in child maltreatment. *Journal of Marriage and the Family, 45:* 773–83.

Gelles, R. (1973) Child abuse as psychopathology: a sociological critique and reformulation. *American Journal of Orthopsychiatry, 43:* 611–21.

Gelles, R. (1978) Violence toward children in the United States. *American Journal of Orthopsychiatry, 48:* 580–92.

Gelles, R. (1979) *Family Violence.* Sage, London.

Gelles, R. & Cornell, C.P. (1983) International perspectives on child abuse. *Child Abuse and Neglect, 7:* 375–86.

George, C. & Main, M. (1979) Social interactions of young abused children: approach, avoidance and aggression. *Child Development, 50:* 306–18.

Gil, D. (1970) *Violence Against Children: Physical Child Abuse in the United States.* Harvard University Press, Cambridge.

Gil, D. (1975) Unravelling child abuse. *American Journal of Orthopsychiatry, 45:* 346–56.

Gil, D. 1979) *Child Abuse and Violence.* AMS, New York.

Gonzalez-Pardo, L. & Thomas, M. (1977) Child abuse and neglect: epidemiology in Kansas. *Journal of the Kansas Medical Society, 78;* 65–69.

Gray, J.D. *et al.* (1979) Prevention and prediction of child abuse and neglect. *Journal of Social Issues, 35:* 127–39.

Green, A.H. *et al.* (1974) Child abuse: pathological syndrome of family interaction. *American Journal of Psychiatry, 131:* 882–86.

Green, A.H. *et al.* (1980) Psychopathological assessment of child-abusing, neglecting and normal mothers. *Journal of Nervous and Mental Diseases, 168* (6): 356–60.

Hall, M.H. (1972) Non-accidental injuries in children. *Royal Society of Health Annual Congress Papers, 79:* 97–102.

Helfer, R. (1982) A review of the literature on the prevention of child abuse and neglect. *Child Abuse and Neglect, 6:* 251–61.

Helfer, R. *et al.* (1977) *Manual for the use of the Michigan Screening Profile of Parenting.* Michigan State University, East Lansing.

Howells, J.G. (1975) Ill-health and child abuse. *Lancet, 2* (7932): 454.

Hyman, C.A. (1978) Some characteristics of abusing families reported to the NSPCC. *British Journal of Social Work, 8:* 31–36.

Ikeda, Y. (1982) A short introduction to child abuse in Japan. *Child Abuse and Neglect, 6:* 423–31.

Jameson, P.A. & Schellenbach, C.J. (1977) Sociological and psychological factors in the backgrounds of male and female perpetrators of child abuse. *Child Abuse and Neglect, 1:* 77–83.

Jobling, M. (1978) Child abuse: the historical and sociological context. In: Carver, V. (ed), *Child Abuse.* Open University Press, Milton Keynes.

Johnson, B. & Morse, H.A. (1968) Injured children and their parents. *Children, 15:* 147–52.

Kadushin, A. & Martin, J.A. (1981) *Child Abuse: An Interactional Event.* Columbia University Press, New York.

Kellmer-Pringle, M. (1980) Towards the prevention of child abuse. In Frude, N. (ed.), *Psychological Approaches to Child Abuse.* Batsford, London.

Kempe, C.H., Silverman, F.N., Steele, B.F., Droegenmueller, W. & Silver, H.K. (1962) The battered child syndrome. *Journal of the American Medical Association, 181:* 17–24.

Kessler, M. & Albee, G.W. (1975) Primary prevention. *Annual Reviews of Psychology, 26:* 557–569.

Kinard, E.M. & Klerman, L.V. (1980) Teenage parenting and child abuse: are they related? *American Journal of Orthopsychiatry, 50* (3): 481–88.

Kline, D.F. (1977) Educational and psychological problems of abused children. *Child Abuse and Neglect, 1:* 301–07.

Korbin, J. (1981) *Child Abuse and Neglect: Cross-cultural Perspectives.* University of California Press, Berkeley.

Kuhn, T. (1962) *The Structure of Scientific Revolutions.* University of Chicago Press, Chicago.

Lahey, B.B. *et al.* (1984) Parenting behavior and emotional status of physically abusive mothers. *Journal of Consulting and Clinical Psychology, 52:* 1062–71.

Lesnik-Oberstein, M. *et al.* (1982) Research in the Netherlands on a theory of child abuse: a preliminary report. *Child Abuse and Neglect, 6:* 199–206.

Leventhal, J.M. (1982) Research strategies and methodologic standards in studies of risk factors for child abuse. *Child Abuse and Neglect, 6:* 113–23.

Lewis, D.O. *et al.* (1979) Delinquents: psychiatric, neurological, psychological and abuse factors. *Journal of the American Academy of Child Psychiatry, 18:* 307–19.

Light, R.J. (1973) Abuse and neglected children in America: a study of alternative policies. *Harvard Educational Review, 43* (4): 556–98.

Loening, W.E.K. (1981) Child abuse among the Zulus: a people in cultural transition. *Child Abuse and Neglect, 5:* 3–7.

Lynch, M. (1975) Ill health and child abuse. *Lancet, 2* (7928): 317–19.

Lynch, M. & Roberts, J. (1977) Prediction of child abuse — signs of bonding failure in the maternity hospital. *British Medical Journal, 1:* 624–26.

Maroulis, H. (1979) Child abuse: the Greek scene. *Child Abuse and Neglect, 3:* 185–90.

Martin, H.P. & Beezley, P. (1977) Behavioral observations of abused children. *Developmental Medicine and Child Neurology, 19:* 373–87.

Martin, H.P. *et al.* (1974) The development of abused children. In: Schulman, I. (ed.), *Advances in Pediatrics. Volume 21.* Year Book Medical Publishers, Chicago.

Morse, C. *et al* (1970) A three-year follow-up of abused and neglected children. *American Journal of Diseases of Childhood, 120:* 439–46.

NSPCC (1985) *Annual Report 1985.* National Society for the Prevention of Cruelty to Children, London.

Newberger, E.H. & Hyde, J.N. (1975) Child abuse: principles and implications of current pediatric practice. *Pediatric Clinics of North America, 22* (3): 695–715.

Nwako, F. (1974) Child abuse syndrome in Nigeria. *International Surgery, 59:* 613–15.

Okeahialam, T.C. (1984) Child abuse in Nigeria. *Child Abuse and Neglect, 8:* 69–73.

Olds, D. (1978) Investigating the prevention of health and developmental problems in children. In: Garbarino, J. & Stocking, S. (eds.), *Supporting Families and Protecting Children.* Center for the Study of Youth Development, Boys Town.

Orme, T.C. & Rimmer, J. (1981) Alcoholism and child abuse: a review. *Journal of Studies on Alcohol, 42:* 273–87.

Ounsted, C. *et al.* (1974) Aspects of bonding failure: the psychopathology and psychotherapeutic treatment of families of battered children. *Developmental Medicine and Child Neurology, 16* (4): 447–56.

Parke, R.D. & Collmer, C.W. (1975) Child abuse: an interdisciplinary analysis. In: Hetherington, E. *et al.* (eds.), *Review of Child Development Research. Vol. 5.* University of Chicago Press, Chicago.

Pelton, L.H. (1978) Child abuse and neglect: the myth of classlessness. *American Journal of Orthopsychiatry, 48:* 608–17.

Pietrse, J.J. (1977) The confidential doctor in the Netherlands. *Child Abuse and Neglect, 1:* 187–94.

Radbill, S.X. (1980) Children in a world of violence: a history of child abuse. In: Kempe, C.H. & Helfer, R.E. (eds.), *The Battered Child.* University of Chicago Press, Chicago.

Roberts, J. *et al.* (1976) Abused children and their siblings: a teacher's view. *Therapeutic Education, 6:* 25–31.

Sameroff, A.J. (1975) Early influences on development: fact or fancy? *Merrill Palmer Quarterly, 21:* 276–94.

Sameroff, A.J. & Chandler, M.J. (1975) Reproductive risk and the continuum of caretaking responsibility. In: Horowitz, F.D. et al. *Reviews of Child Development Research. Volume 4.* University of Chicago Press, Chicago.

Sandgrund, A. *et al.* (1974) Child abuse and mental retardation: a problem of cause and effect. *American Journal of Mental Deficiency, 79:* 327–30.

Scott, P.D. (1973) Fatal battered baby cases. *Medicine, Science and the Law, 13:* 197–206.

Sills, J.A. *et al.* (1977) Non-accidental injury: a two year study in central Liverpool. *Developmental Medicine and Child Neurology, 19:* 26–33.

Smith, S. & Deasy, P. (1977) Child abuse in Ireland. *Journal of the Irish Medical Association, 70* (3): 65–79.

Smith, S. & Hanson, R. (1974) 135 battered children: a medical and psychological study. *British Medical Journal, 2:* 666–70.

Smith, S. & Hanson, R. (1975) Interpersonal relationships and child rearing practices in 214 parents of battered children. *British Journal of Psychiatry, 127:* 513–25.

Soumenkoff, G. *et al.* (1982) A coordinated attempt for prevention of child abuse at the antenatal care level. *Child Abuse and Neglect, 6:* 87–94.

Spinetta, J.J. & Rigler, D. (1972) The child abusing parent: a psychological review. *Pyschological Bulletin, 77:* 296–304.

Starr, R.H. (1979) Child abuse. *American Psychologist, 34* (10): 872–78.

Starr, R.H. (1982) A research-based approach to the prediction of child abuse. In: Starr, R.H. (ed.), *Child Abuse Prediction: Policy Implications.* Ballinger, Cambridge.

Steele, B.F. (1970) Parental abuse of infants and small children. In: Anthony, E.J. & Benedek, T. (eds.), *Parenthood: Its Psychology and Psychopathology.* Churchill, Edinburgh.

Steele, B.F. & Pollock, C.B. (1974) A psychiatric study of parents who abuse infants and small children. In: Helfer, R.E. & Kempe, C.H. (eds.), *The Battered Child.* University of Chicago Press, Chicago.

Stein, A.H. & Friedrich, L.K. (1975) Impact of television on children and youth. In: Hetherington, E.M. *et al.* (eds.), *Review of Child Development Research. Vol. 5.* University of Chicago Press, Chicago.

Steinmetz, S. & Straus, M. (1974) *Violence in the Family.* Dodd Mead, New York.

Stern, L. (1973) Prematurity as a factor in child abuse. *Hospital Practice, 8:* 117–23.

Straus, M. *et al.* (1980) *Behind Closed Doors.* Doubleday, Garden City.

Sweet, J.J. & Resick, P.A. (1979) The maltreatment of children: a review of theories and research. *Journal of Social Issues, 35* (2): 40–59.

Tauber, E. *et al.* (1977) Child ill-treatment as considered by the Italian criminal and civil codes. *Child Abuse and Neglect, 1:* 149–52.

Thompson, E.P. (1968) *The Making of the English Working Class.* Penguin, Harmondsworth.

Toro, P.A. (1982) Developmental aspects of child abuse: a review. *Child Abuse and Neglect, 6:* 423–31.

Vasta, R. (1982) Physical child abuse: a dual-component analysis. *Developmental Review, 2:* 125–49.

Vesterdal, J. (1977) Handling of child abuse in Denmark. *Child Abuse and Neglect, 1:* 193–98.

Westermeyer, J. & Bearman, J. (1973) A proposed social indicator system for alcohol-related problems. *Preventive Medicine, 2:* 438–44.

Wilson, C. & Orford, J. (1978) Children of alcoholics: report of a preliminary study and comments on the literature. *Journal of Studies on Alcohol, 39:* 121–42.

Wolfe, D.A. (1985) Child-abusive parents: an empirical review and analysis. *Psychological Bulletin, 97* (3): 462–82.

World Health Organization (1984) *World Health Statistics Annual.* WHO, Geneva.

Wright, L. (1976) The 'slick but sick' syndrome as a personality component of parents of battered children. *Journal of Clinical Psychology, 32:* 41–45.

Young, L.R. (1964) *Wednesday's Children: a Study of Neglect and Abuse.* McGraw-Hill, New York.

Zenz, G. (1978) Legal aspects of child abuse in the practice of custody courts in the Federal Republic of Germany. In: Eekelaar, J.M. & Katz, N.S. (eds.), *Family Violence: an International and Interdisciplinary Study.* Butterworths, Toronto.

Ziegert, K.A. (1983) The Swedish prohibition of corporal punishment: a preliminary report. *Journal of Marriage and the Family, 45:* 917–26.

EXPLOITATION OF WORKING CHILDREN: SITUATION ANALYSES AND APPROACHES TO IMPROVING THEIR CONDITIONS

U. S. Naidu*

INTRODUCTION

Children of under 15 years working for economic gain are found all over the world, in pockets of poverty in industrialized countries, and in developing countries in very large numbers. There is concern for these children because most of them work for their survival and to support their families.

Child labour obviously does not feature here as a part of socialization and an experience that promotes growth and development. This paper focuses on the negative aspects of child labour and examines some approaches to the improvement of conditions of working children and their protection from exploitation.

Causes of Child Labour

Poverty and inequity are the major causes of child labour. A number of studies (United Nations 1982, Dogramaci, 1985, Naidu, 1985) have indicated that development is inversely related to the incidence of child labour. In other words, it is in the countries, states and districts with high illiteracy rates and backwardness in economic development, combined with poor environmental resources, that the problem of child labour is found.

The prevalence of child labour can be explained by multiple factors — psychological, social, cultural, economic and political. It is difficult to separate the contribution that each makes to its prevalence or perpetuation. All are interlinked, and consequently the impact of one can be studied only in relation to that of the others.

Psychological, social and cultural factors

Child labour depends upon normative attitudes towards children in society, the culturally determined roles and functions of children, the values by which the activities of children are judged, and the nature of the socialization process. In industrialized countries there is general disapproval of participation of school-age children in the formal labour force. The participation of children in housework is approved, by parents at least. In many countries, participation in various types of economic activities from an early age is considered an essential part of socialization.

The prevailing modes of domestic organization and systems of kinship and marriage also affect child labour. What children must do is influenced by what the system of kinship considers the rights and obligations of children. In some places the delegation of aspects of parental roles, and the institutionalized practice of fostering of children by non-parental kin, involve widespread

---

* Professor and Head, Unit for Child and Youth Research, Tata Institute of Social Sciences, P.B. 8313, Deonar, Bombay 400 088, India.

transfers of the obligation to train and maintain children, and the right to enjoy the services of the young. Such practices may involve an element of apprenticeship and specialist training.

Another example of the independent effects of these factors is the attribution of sex roles among children. Some aspects of these roles clearly consist of preparation for the adult sexual division of labour. Thus it seems almost universal that child care and housework fall more to females than to males, in keeping with the traditional view of the domestic role of women.

In Indian society, although it is changing slowly, there still exists a strict compartmentalization of groups of people on the basis of a caste hierarchy. The traditional occupational roles for each of the caste groups are defined. According to such definitions Brahmins belong to the priestly caste, Kshatriya to the warrior caste, Vaishya to business, and Shudra to service caste groups. For their source of income both Brahmins and Shudras depend to a large extent upon the middle caste-groups. However, there is a significant difference between the two groups in their social status. Brahmins hold the supreme position in society, whereas Shudras are on the lowest rung of the social ladder.

A series of social reforms designed to narrow the social inequality have not achieved their objectives. In general, only the upper caste and class groups have taken advantage of education and, as a result, Brahmins have slowly moved away from their traditional roles. Urbanization and industrialization have reinforced this move by attracting large numbers of Brahmins to urban areas to man the new offices. The lower-caste groups could not avail of this opportunity. Their lowly position in society made them feel inferior and this deterred them from seeking education. In the process, the lower-caste groups, which remained uneducated, became economically more dependent upon the middle castes. However, there is much more variability in the extent to which girls work outside the home, which cannot be fully explained by socioeconomic factors. For instance, Islamic traditions restrict the participation of females in the labour force; indeed, in Arab countries the prevalence of restrictions on female activity, presumably reflecting cultural orthodoxy rather than economic need, is statistically associated with a lower participation of females in the labour force (Azzam, 1979).

The psychological, social and cultural factors are also interdependent with the economic system within which they operate. For example, at a broader level, the roles of children are associated with the values which parents attach to children, with the images of the future which parents hold, and with the objectives underlying particular levels of fertility. Although parents give many reasons for having children, the work of children, domestic or otherwise, recurs frequently. Parents see the birth of children as a means of adding to the household labour force. In their view, the child comes into the world with one mouth to eat and two hands to work. Of course, they see children also as providing happiness, companionship, and psychological satisfaction. However, these benefits can be obtained with two or three children. The motivation to have more has underlying economic reasons.

High birth rates in developing countries, with a marked fall in mortality rates in early life, have resulted in the survival of larger numbers of children. The poor have been affected adversely by this demographic change. The proportion of children aged up to 14 years to the population in the 15–59 age group is higher among the poor than among the better-off. Poor families are consequently handicapped in having relatively few employable persons in the prescribed working age. There is a heavy pressure of dependency, mostly of young children, on poor families, and this perpetuates child labour among them.

Economic and political factors

Stronger than tradition or values is the effect of poverty on the prevalence and perpetuation of child labour. The economic reforms aimed at reducing economic inequality among social groups have in some ways proved counterproductive. In India and other countries of South-East Asia, land reform was attempted as a means of reducing poverty and unemployment. The official policies of low taxation of agricultural incomes and assets, and subsidization of modernizing measures, combined with the wealthy farmers' advantage of being able to invest finance, encouraged large landowners to take more interest in farm management than they had taken. They took back the land which had been leased out to small farmers or landless labourers. Thus, the traditional means of viable self-employment which had been created by the leasing system were, in effect, either withdrawn or made less available to a certain proportion of rural households. Further, technological changes in agriculture made the management of small farms very uneconomic. So-called 'appropriate technology' favoured wealthy farmers and harmed small tenant operators. Some self-employed farmers began to search for wage employment. Thus, the land reforms displaced a significant proportion of population from self-employment to wage employment, and from the small land-owning to the landless class. The result is massive immigration of the lower class from villages.

Thus, any examination of psychological, social and cultural factors of child labour should consider their interaction with economic and political processes.

Magnitude of the Problem

Since in most countries child labour is not given legal sanction, children work in the 'informal sector'; therefore, it is very difficult to discover the precise number of children at work. Various authorities have attempted global estimates of the number of working children in the world. In 1979 the International Labour Organization (ILO) estimated the number at 52 million, but, in 1983, the Director General of ILO indicated that this was 'a conservative estimate'. Recently a United Nations (UN 1982) report gave the figure of 145 million working children between the ages of 10 and 14 years. This figure seems realistic. A picture of the number of children in the labour force in a few selected countries is given in Tables I and II. Although these figures are based on uneven data, it is clear that child labour is concentrated in developing countries.

Children's Occupations

Children are mostly employed in the informal sector, and in almost all the activities in which adults are employed in this sector, mainly agriculture, fishing, forestry, plantation work, the hand-loom industry, the construction of buildings and roads, and match-box manufacture. They are also employed in domestic service, and in hotels, restaurants and canteens. Some are engaged in the trash-recycling business, selling such items as artificial jewellery, vegetables, fruits, snacks and newspapers.

Table 1. Population under the age of 15 years and rate of activity, by region and sex, 1975

| | Population under the age of 15 years | | | | |
| | (thousands) | | (percentage) | | |
Region	Boys	Girls	Boys	Girls	Average rate by boys and girls
Africa	88965	88354	6.8	4.0	5.4
Latin America	69016	67215	3.5	1.2	2.4
North America	30794	29572	0.8	0.4	0.6
East Asia South-East Asia }	444234	424490	5.2	4.0	4.7
Europe	57831	55261	0.8	0.6	0.7
Oceania	3431	3272	2.5	1.9	2.2
USSR	33486	32263	0.0	0.0	0.0
	727757	700428	4.5	3.2	3.8

Source: ILO, Yearbook of Labour Statistics, 1978 and Bureau of Statistics and Special Studies.

Table 2. Number and percentage of boys and girls aged 10 to 14 in the labour force in selected countries, 1975

Country	Boys		Girls		Total	
	Number (thousands)	Percentage	Number (thousands)	Percentage	Number (thousands)	Percentage
Brazil	1054	15.8	382	5.8	1436	10.8
China	5397	12.1	4128	9.6	9525	10.9
Egypt	426	18.2	101	4.5	527	11.5
Hungary	2	0.6	4	1.3	6	1.0
India	7620	19.4	7537	20.7	15157	20.0
Indonesia	1425	16.5	1048	12.5	2473	14.5
Italy	70	3.1	44	2.0	114	2.6
Mexico	390	10.0	91	2.4	481	6.3
Mozambique	220	41.8	77	14.5	297	28.1
Peru	44	4.6	40	4.3	84	4.5
Sweden	2	0.6	1	0.3	3	0.4
Thailand	623	23.0	730	27.7	1353	25.4
United States of America	221	2.1	106	1.1	327	1.6
United Republic of Tanzania	334	35.9	223	23.9	557	29.9

Source: M.C. McHale and J. McHale, *Children in the World* (Washington) D.C. Population Reference Bureau, 1979), p. 65.

Forms of Exploitation of Working Children

Children have always worked. In the best circumstances, work prepares them for productive adult life. However, a balance of work, learning and play should be maintained and this is not always done. Child work becomes exploitation if it prevents access to education, leaves no time for recreation, or is hazardous to their health.

Exploitative child labour implies the premature assumption of adult roles, working long hours for low wages, damage to physical and psychosocial health, and denial of opportunities for education and recreation.

Child exploitation takes many forms. The spectrum of exploitation may be studied from various viewpoints. The presence of a family is one of the highly significant criteria for examining its prevalent forms. Family support for children may be full or partial, continuous or occasional. Working children without family support are more vulnerable to exploitation than are those with full or occasional family support.

Bonded labour is prevalent among landless peasants. A peasant family commits to its landlord certain labour services in repayment of debt. One form of bonded labour is the pledging of children to landlords for their whole lives as part payment of family debt. Another is to send children from rural areas with middle men to work in child-labour-intensive trade centres, for example, to work at carpet-weaving. Children are enslaved to work in such trades. Yet another form is to force children to migrate for employment and live with their employers.

EFFECTS OF EMPLOYMENT ON CHILDREN

Health problems

The health of exploited working children is endangered by work under conditions that are hazardous to health. Working children come from the poorer segments of the population and thus start with poor health from malnutrition and insufficient intake of energy. Their work then increases their nutritional needs, which they are mostly unable to meet, and thus, their health is likely to be damaged still more as a result of having to go into employment at an early age.

Largely, the health consequences of child labour have not been investigated. The World Health Organization has made pioneer efforts by convening multidisciplinary meetings and training workshops on research methodologies, and by sponsoring research into effects on health of child labour in developing countries.

Malnutrition: Normal growth spurts during puberty and adolescence are adversely affected by poor nutrient intake and increased manual work. Studies have shown that malnutrition in early childhood continuing into adolescence adversely affects children's work capacity by its influence on body weight (Satyanarayan *et al.*, 1979, Naidu & Parasuraman, 1985).

Communicable diseases: Children at work come into close contact with infectious cases of tuberculosis. Severe malnutrition, anaemia, hard labour, fatigue and inadequate sleep increase their susceptibility to infectious diseases. Children are given the dirtiest jobs, avoided by adults, such as trash collection from garbage spots, with maximum exposure to insanitary conditions. Children at work may be exposed to toxic substances. The effects of lead poisoning have been documented, in zari brocade workers, who inhale very fine particles of zari (Banerji, 1979). The consequences of work environments, poor background nutrition and higher exposure to communicable diseases by working children as compared with non-working children needs further scientific investigation.

Occupational hazards: Children's health may be impaired because of working in particular occupations with poisoning from welding, byssinosis from textile manufacturing, and venereal diseases from prostitution. The impairments may appear at the beginning of work or become manifest only much later. Injuries are immediate. Their association with work is, therefore unequivocal. Many diseases which can take decades to become manifest are occupational, such as asbestosis, chronic cadmium toxicity and certain cancers. Hence, it is not easy to convince the people about the long-term adverse effects of some occupations in which children are engaged.

Psychosocial hazards: Childhood is the stage of personality formation. Children in exploitative work are likely to suffer permanent adverse psychosocial consequences of the physical and emotional stress of work combined with the denial of opportunity to play, explore the world, and interact fully with other children, and physical and emotional abuse and neglect, separation from family, monotony and the burdens of premature responsibility. A recent study in Bombay (Naidu and Parasuraman, 1985) reported that working children are frustrated, suffer from role-conflicts, and have low occupationai, income and educational aspirations.

Effects on education: For a detailed assessment of the effects of child labour on the children's education, statistics are not available. However, according to some estimates few working children attend school, fewer complete primary education and only a very small number can combine earning and learning. Most working children are illiterate. Long hours of work reduce the possibility of any kind of schooling. In most countries schools operate during the day and full-time. Poor families cannot afford school fees, books, or uniforms. The curricula of conventional schools are unsuitable and irrelevant for the children of poverty groups. Since certification from schools and colleges are linked with employment opportunities, such deprivation bars these children from any chance of better employment in life.

In some cases, instead of schooling, children are placed in employment units as apprentices. In principle this could compensate for long working hours or lack of schooling but, in practice, the apprenticeship of children has itself become a severe form of exploitation. Children are put to apprenticeship for years to avoid the payment of wages and the provision of other facilities, or they are used as servants for tasks unrelated to the trade for which they are being trained.

Effects of working conditions. Children work in rural, urban and metropolitan areas, but mostly in rural areas. The conditions of work in urban and metropolitan areas are very different from those in rural areas. One critical variable in children's work settings is the degree of family support. As long as children work as part of a family group, the work is likely to be adapted to their physical capacity (Gore, 1985). Parents are unlikely to, or will not, insist that children do work that they are physically unable to do. However, young children working in cities enter into a very different type of employer-employee relationship, which can give rise to a variety of exploitative practices. One aspect of exploitation is that the children work much beyond their physical capacity; another is low wages; and still another is the bonding of the child for certain types of activities which adults would object to doing.

Typically, child labour is characterized by unhygienic conditions, long hours of work, low wages in relation to the amount of work, no health or medical-care benefits, working in poor ventilation, and working without any paid leave. However, there is a concentration of children in some of the more hazardous occupations, such as carpet-weaving, the match-box industry, textiles, the slate-pencil industry, and the construction industry.

Approaches used to Improve the Conditions of Working Children and Protect them from Exploitation

Four major approaches have been taken to deal with child labour and protect children from exploitation. They are: (1) legislative protective measures; (2) the area development approach; (3) ameliorative services for children; and (4) changing nature of work to suit the child's stage of development.

Legislative measures for protection

The International Labour Organization has been for decades one of the most outspoken advocates of legislation for the protection of children from exploitation and the prohibition of child labour. The issues on which it has promoted legislation have been (a) setting the minimum age of 15 years for entry into employment; (b) banning the employment of children in hazardous conditions; (c) improving working conditions — for example, equal pay for equal work, weekly rest-days, and medical care. Some countries have ratified ILO conventions on these issues but many have not, and in many cases those that have done so have not implemented them fully.

Thus, although legal protection is a useful instrument for dealing with the worst child-labour abuses, legislation to abolish child labour and to protect children from exploitation would not in itself be the solution of the problem. Legislation provides a frame, but its implementation needs other developmental supports.

The area development approach

Under this approach an area is selected which has a high concentration of child labour. It then receives multiple developmental inputs on the assumption that children will benefit from the general development of the area. Some services are designated for the working children. One such unique experiment began in 1984 at Sivakasi, Sattur and Vembakottari Blocks in Tamil Nadu, India, as a collaborative effort of the Tamil Nadu State Government, the United Nations Children's Fund (UNICEF) and the owners of match factories. The Ministry of Social Welfare is the nodal ministry for the project and it coordinates the participation of eight departments from other ministries — the departments of public health and preventive medicine, medical services, water supply and drainage, education, labour through a nutrition project which it sponsors, applied research, rural development, and local bodies. The project has been planned, discussed, revised and modified to meet the challenges of the field. Such experimental projects are welcomed as systematic efforts for the protection of children from exploitation and ultimately the abolition of child labour.

Ameliorative services for working children

This approach has focused on providing working children with such basic services as health care, nutrition and education. Some efforts have been made, particularly by non-governmental organizations, to provide such services with or without government support. Most of the programmes are limited to certain parts of a few cities and there are few beneficiaries in proportion to the number who could benefit.

Changing the nature of work to suit the development of working children

The object of this approach is to change the nature of children's work so that it would conduce to their development instead of hindering it. In India the Ministry of Labour has sponsored a few such experimental programmes in metropolitan areas and small towns. The approach appears promising. As a result employers hire youngsters, not because they are cheap labour, but because they are dependable and productive workers. The programmes are managed by non-governmental organizations. Children are being helped to grow and develop by intervening on their behalf with their employers and their families.

STRATEGIES FOR DEALING WITH THE EXPLOITATION OF CHILD LABOUR

Multi-level interventions

Interventions that will improve the condition of working children, prevent their exploitation, and result in the abolition of child labour in developing countries will need to be made at various levels, namely, at those of government, community, family, employers and working children themselves (Table 3).

Multisectoral approach to the problem

Child labour is a complex problem which needs an intersectoral approach involving the sectors of health, labour, agriculture, education, industry, rural, economic planning, and social welfare. Without such an approach the full social and health impact of child labour escapes the awareness of many sectors and its appropriate priority for all sectors.

Integrated developmental services for working children

The objective of such services is to alleviate the hardships to which working children are often exposed and to improve their working conditions and future possibilities by the provision of subsidized food, minimum levels of health

Table 3. Intervention levels according to settings of child work*

	Suggested Intervention Levels				
Settings of Child Work	Govt.	Comm.	Fam.	Emp.	W. Child
1. *Within the family* (Unpaid)					
i) Domestic tasks — cleaning, child-care, cooking, washing clothes, fetching water, etc.	*		*		
ii) Agricultural and pastoral tasks — ploughing, harvesting, herding, etc.	*	*	*		
iii) Cottage industries — leather-work, wood-work, various traditional household occupations	*	*	*		*
2. *With the family but outside the home*					
i) Bonded	*		*	*	
ii) Agricultural and pastoral work					
a. Migrant labour	*		*	*	*
b. Local agricultural labour	*	*	*	*	*
iii) Domestic service	*		*	*	
iv) Construction work	*	*	*	*	*
v) Rag-picking/recycling trash business			*	*	*
3. *Outside the Family*					
A. *Employed by others*					
i) Bonded	*	*	*	*	*
ii) Apprentices	*			*	*
iii) Skilled traders — carpet-weaving, brass and copper work, embroidery, etc.	*	*	*	*	*
iv) Manufacturing units — plastics, glass, slate-pencil, artificial jewellery, match stick making, etc.	*	*	*	*	*
v) Repair shops Garages for cars, scooter, cycle repairs				*	*
vi) Domestic service				*	*
vii) Establishments e.g., shops, restaurants				*	*
viii) Begging	*	*	*	*	*
ix) Prostitution	*	*	*	*	*
B. *Self-employed* e.g "shoe-shining", selling vegetables, fruits, snacks, artificial jewellery, newspapers; rag picking, etc.		*	*		*

Notes: Govt. = Government
Comm. = Community
Fam. = Family
Emp. = Employer
W. Child = Working child

* This table refers to conditions in India. The framework may be adapted to those of other countries.

protection, education, and improvements in the conditions of the work-place. As far as possible, such services should be provided at or near the work-place, and in the case of health care the possibility of using special mobile health services should be explored. Since evening classes may impose an additional burden on already overworked children, literacy and related activities may need to be carried out during the day, often during working hours.

Urgent action for relieving children working in hazardous conditions

Strict measures are needed without further delay to relieve the children working in conditions that have direct risks to their health and life; examples are mining, the slate-pencil industry, carpet-weaving, textiles, and construction work, to name but a few. Modalities of action can be devised with the help of experts, officials, employers and parents of the working children.

Orienting the service sector to the needs of working children

The staff of hospitals, dispensaries and clinics should be asked to record the work status of children, when they present for the treatment of any disease or injury. Preventive social medicine staff and other community health workers should be trained and made responsible for working children in their programmes. Child health services should be provided at children's work-places as well as at their homes and schools. School teachers need to be made aware of the conditions of working children so that they may be responsive to their needs.

Adult employment guarantee

The emphasis has to be on fuller employment of adults in the family, with adequate wages, so that children may enjoy their childhood. This would promote the withdrawal of children from the labour force.

Reduction of infant mobility

Efforts have to be directed towards reducing infant mortality, which would encourage parents to believe that every single child born in a family has a high chance of survival. Thus, parents could plan to have fewer children and be secure from the anxiety of losing children in their early years of life.

Provision of day-care centres cum schools

The provision of day-care centres cum schools would greatly benefit young girls who work and when not at work have to mind siblings to relieve their mothers for work. It would serve two purposes: a reduction in the drop-out rate of girls in schools, and an increase in the school enrollment of girls from the population of working children.

Meaningful education cum vocational training

Working children and other children from poverty groups have clearly shown the irrelevance of conventional education in their lives, by their non-enrollment in schools and by dropping out. It is important not only to provide for their access to education but also to change the content of the education and methods of teaching so as to make it relevant for them.

Development of backward areas

The prevalence of child labour in any area is inversely related with development. General development of backward areas, and improvement in the economic conditions of marginal farmers, landless labourers in particular, would have the effect of reducing the numbers of child workers. This strategy would attack the problem at its root by improving the conditions of the sector of the population which is prone to migration owing to poverty.

The role of Non-Governmental Organizations

Non-governmental organizations (NGOs) have a crucial role to play in the prevention of exploitation of working children, in the provision of developmental services to them, and in the abolition of child labour. It is clear from Table 3 that interventions have to be made at the levels of government, community, family, employers, and the working children themselves. At times governments may not recognize the problem of child labour, may suppress information about it, or may even deliberately or otherwise perpetuate child labour. In such circumstances NGOs can function as a pressure group on governments. Communities and families may become resigned to poverty, helplessness and lack of power; NGOs may function as catalysts to build up their strength. At times, employers in the unorganized sector, where most of the children are working, form an organization, and this may give NGOs opportunities to intervene with them to prevent the exploitation of working children. There are some cooperative employers who can be approached easily, and children can be helped to utilize basic services. Children at work have assumed premature adulthood: they need not only to be educated and counselled but also to be relieved of the burden they carry prematurely. Thus, NGOs can play an active developmental role at macro- and micro-levels to reach this unreached group of children so that their right to childhood will be restored to them.

References

Azzam, H. *The participation of the Arab woman in the labour force: development factors and policies.* (World Employment Programme Research Working Paper), Geneva, International Labour Organization, 1979.

Banerji, S. *Child labour in India.* London: Anti-Slavery Society, 1979.

Dogramaci, I. Child Labour: An Overview. In: P.M. Shah (ed.), *Child labour: a threat to health and development,* Geneva, Defence for Children International, 1985.

Gore, M.S. Opening address, In: U.S. Naidu & K.R. Kapadia (eds.), *Child labour and health: problems and prospects,* Tata Institute of Social Sciences, Bombay, 1985.

Naidu, U.S. Health problems of working children — some issues in planning long term care. In: U.S. Naidu & K.R. Kapadia (eds.), *Child labour and health: problems and prospects,* Tata Institute of Social Sciences, Bombay, 1985.

Naidu, U.S. & Parasuraman, S. *Health situation of working children in Greater Bombay,* (Study sponsored by WHO, Geneva), Tata Institute of Social Sciences, Bombay, 1985 (Mimeo).

Satyanarayan, K. et al. Body size and work output, *Am. J. Clin. Nut.* 30: 322 (1977).

United Nations, *Exploitation of child labour* (A. Bouhdiba), New York, 1982.

LATIN AMERICA: CHILD ABUSE AND VAGRANCY

F. Reyes Romero*

The urban population of Latin America is increasing and its problems are compounded by its numbers in spite of the efforts of various types of government — dictatorships of the left and right, bourgeois democracies and peoples democracies; 280 million people are caught up in a process of relentless social change and are growing poorer every day, although their lands remain rich. The socioeconomic, political and cultural conditions in which they live generate an abusive environment, which produces a harsh and violent childhood among the lower social strata, with few positive rewards.

Child vagrancy is on the increase in Colombia, Mexico and Brazil, and in the central and crowded areas of all the cities of Latin America. The "poverty toll" — children and adults or adults with babies in their arms haunting street corners near traffic lights to beg from motorists is now a common sight.

In Central America, Colombia and Peru children of 11–14 years are recruited into guerrilla groups and this imposes upon them a whole process of adaptation and exertion out of all proportion to their age and physical strength in carrying out the missions imposed by their leaders. In Chile, Argentina and Uruguay adults have "disappeared", leaving their 'orphaned" children with serious maladjustment problems; children have also disappeared. In Colombia an increasing number of children are being kidnapped from their homes throughout the country, at the rate of almost one a week.

Some of the children on the streets have street occupations — boot-blacks, car-minders, or touting cigarettes, sweets, marijuana or bazuco (cocaine), or accompanying their parents in hawking food, clothes or other articles. Other children have taken permanently to begging. Many have become involved in the sex market; boys and girls are being drawn into child prostitution and child pornography.

The life of the groups from which these children come is a constant struggle for survival, and this complicates any approaches by governments or by nongovernmental agencies. This is the result of a structural situation common to the whole of Latin America. The most dramatic cases of battering are to be found mostly in the marginal sectors of the population and usually reach the casualty departments of the children's hospitals under some other cover, nearly always in the guise of accidents.

Abuse and Vagrancy

Any battering or other type of abuse that occurs in the middle and upper social classes is usually dealt with in private consultations or by the social security service, which helps to mask the real situation and contributes to underreporting. However, the vast majority of the people are in the lower social classes and they are commonly found in the unplanned slum or shanty settlements known as "tugurios" or "favelas", "villas miseria", "poblaciones callampa" or "pueblos

---

* Director, Medical Care, Ministry of Health, Calle 16 numero 7-39, Bogota D.E., Colombia

jóvenes". This is where the drama of disruption and loss of parental authority is played out day after day by country people as they reach the cities for the first time with their familes. It is where their distress is compounded as men fail to find work and see the end of their role as father and head of the family, fulfilling an economic responsibility, and are forced to accept the meagre income raised by their children from casual work or by their wives from domestic service. This starts the process; the lack of adequate or even basic shelter is compounded by the lack of water supply and sewage disposal systems and the high cost of food and transport. But something more is lost. Family relationships, which were relatively peaceful when they lived in the country, deteriorate into constant strife, which may lead to physical assault, from which children are not spared; one immediate cause is drink, to which the peasants resort to forget their desperate situation and to help overcome the permanent frustration which leads to depression. Lost in this anonymity, the family members individually and the family as a whole are at the mercy of a society that neglects them, gives them no opportunity to work, and provides none of the services which their increasing poverty does not permit them to purchase.

Where sexual abuse is concerned, these are communities where incest and promiscuity are more common than in the better off, and whose values are different. There are also some mentally disordered people whose sexual behaviour is abnormal and who are often responsible for assaults on children under seven. Most of these acts go unpunished, for these marginal groups have little or no police services, no legal assistance to hand, or no access to official protection of any kind.

Abandonment is a widespread form of abuse in Latin America, as evidenced by the presence of child vagrancy in the big cities, a problem which has attracted worldwide attention and has been studied by a number of researchers. In Colombia the phenomenon of child vagrancy — "gamines" — made its appearance many years ago, at the beginning of this century; many studies have been carried out on it, programmes have been established and contacts made with the families and communities from which these children have come. These studies have shown that the type and structure of society is the principal factor in determining the appearance of this form of societal abuse. Quantification of this social phenomenon is difficult since there are several types of child vagrants: those on the streets day and night, those who spend the night there, those who are there in the daytime, those who are there during school holiday periods, and others who spend their lives permanently roaming the larger cities.

In the study by the Colombian Institute of Family Welfare entitled "Child vagrants, their social support and families", published in 1978, physical abuse was found to be the second most important reason for children to leave their homes and swell the ranks of the vagrants. Observations in other countries of Latin America such as Argentina, Chile, Peru, Brazil, Mexico, Ecuador, Uruguay and Venezuela have evidenced the physical abuse experienced by these children in early childhood before they left home, only to be followed by continual ill-treatment at the hands of the police, teachers and other institutional workers and irresponsible adults. The presence of a stepfather in the home may be a barrier to these children's relationship with their mother, who must take transient companions in order to survive, and increases the likelihood of rough treatment. The children have described the physical punishments received at the hands of their own mothers — beating or lashing with belts, cables, sticks, machetes or knives, and their hands, and sometimes even beatings by their own fathers while they were still living at home in the early years. It is common to find children who have been ill-treated by fathers who are alcoholics or drug addicts. The children who have been battered in early childhood readily develop similar behaviour patterns themselves, and these are reinforced in corrective institutions and prisons; thus a generation is produced which is in turn likely to ill-treat their own children or other people with whom they may come into contact in their lives.

The gangs of child vagrants that form to live and sleep on the streets are known as "galladas" and "camadas"; these groups are ruled by the toughest of their members and any informer or "sapo" ("toadies") are severely punished, while the smallest members are treated brutally because they are the most defenceless and have no possible recourse to help.

The number of street girls and vagrant girls is also increasing. Many become pregnant, usually between the ages of 14 and 16 years; their children's environment will be negative in every sense of the word, with ill-treatment by their parents compounded by abuse at the hands of all the other adults with whom they may come into contact. The girls are very soon drawn into child prostitution, now no longer confined to girls, and springing up at or near the night clubs frequented by tourists.

We have found that 90% of child vagrants suffered physical ill-treatment in early childhood, and that this was subsequently reinforced by ill-treatment at the corrective institutions to which they were sent, not only at the hands of teachers but also from the other staff. They have suffered ill-treatment at the hands of the police also, and have thus been subjected to brutality from a whole string of aggressors, with the result that they will in turn retaliate against a society which has always been hostile. Also, they and their siblings have suffered from various degrees of malnutrition, anaemia, acute respiratory infections and acute diarrhoeal diseases; they are particularly prone to accidents from motor vehicles and a variety of other causes; and they show a high prevalence of sexually transmitted diseases, now appearing in both boys and girls.

Despite their experience, however, many of these children have taken advantage of informal educational opportunities and have built up their own philosophy and thought about the problem of ill-treatment; their awareness of the problem has led them to react positively to their own children, thus breaking out of the vicious circle which makes the victims of abuse in turn likely to ill-treat their children.

Colombia

The extreme poverty which extends throughout Latin America is to be seen in Colombia also, and the increase in the urban population — more than 70% — completes the desolate backdrop to the various forms of child abuse. Children are drawn into domestic work from the age of four onwards, and into small family and private industries, where they do heavy work, which in the rural areas consists of agricultural and domestic tasks, and at harvest time the picking and carrying of the crops, especially coffee and cotton. Children have traditionally worked in the coal-mines. One example of this is the Department of Boyacá, where a school census showed that 100% of the children, whose ages ranged between 5 and 15, took part in agricultural work and 50% in mining also.

In 1981, 109 cases of maltreated children were seen at the Hospital de la Misericordia in Bogota, constituting 0.22% of all consultations, with more boys than girls, and with 41% between the ages of five and nine, and 30% between 10 and 14; 93% were from Bogota and 7% from the surrounding rural area. The four most common types of ill-treatment found were: 54% various types of injuries, 25% abandonment with exposure, and the remainder falls and poisonings. The most recent statistics, for January to October 1985, show that accidents were the leading reason for consultation, whereas in previous years they had been in third place. Cases of battering constitute 1% of these accidents.

In a report submitted by the University Hospital of Valle on 43 cases of maltreated children, half were under the age of five years and half between five and 14 (February-August 1984); 8% presented soft-tissue lesions and 16% had severe head injuries or damage to the abdomen or urinary tract.

Analysis of all casualty and outpatient consultations at the Lorencita Villegas de Santos Hospital in Bogota showed that, from January to December 1984, cases of child abuse accounted for 0.10%, and from January to July 1985 for 0.12%, with more girls than boys, and infants as the worst affected group.

In a study of cases referred to the Hospital de le Misericordia in Bogota, parents — mothers and to a less extent, fathers — were responsible for abuse in 76% of 109 cases; in a study of 137 cases undertaken by the Colombian Institute of Family Welfare (1982) to investigate the type of abuse, 73% was found to be physical aggression and 22% sexual abuse. Meanwhile, the Office of Forensic Medicine reported that, of 351 cases of sexual abuse in 1984, 90% involved girls and 10% boys; an earlier study from the children's hospital reported 70% girls and 30% boys.

This problem has been brought to public notice by those in charge of the casualty departments of the Misericordia and the Lorencita Villegas de Santos children's hospitals in Bogota, and the University Hospital of Valle in Cali, and by authors of theses or books on the question, such as *The Drama and Tragedy of Child Workers,* by Roberto Gutiérrez. The Colombian Institute of Family Welfare, whose task it is to undertake action and research to protect children, has put forward a number of solutions, while other institutions, such as IDIPRON — District Institute for the Protection of Children — have organized work-schemes for the victims of maltreatment, which reach out to the family and thus break into the vicious circle of generations of child battering.

CONCLUSION

Some of the observations presented here are based on the author's experience between 1966 and 1969 with 550 middle- and lower-class schoolchildren from the city of Bogota; 1615 Bogota child vagrants from 1970 to 1985; 200 child vagrants from cities other than Bogota, over the same period, as well as 250 from Brazil, Argentina, Chile, Mexico, Peru, Ecuador, Uruguay and Venezuela; and 700 primary-school children from rural areas in 1975.

The author has also followed up 130 cases of child vagrants over the last 15 years, examining their family background, their adaptation to the family environment after they have been at rehabilitation centres, their employment, their health problems, and the extent of violence in their relations with children and other people. The work with child vagrants was at first carried out in their own environment, where methods for approaching and dealing with them were worked out, and then with six- to eight-year-olds in an institution; a group of 30 children received informal education followed by six months' experimental self-responsibility. Also, an experimental teaching programme was carried out with 150 children with the cooperation of trainee teachers and military servicemen. All these experiences have permitted direct and continuous observation of the process of rehabilitation, and the follow-up of 27% of discharged children.

CHILDREN IN WAR: IMPLICATIONS FOR THE HEALTH WORKER IN THE EIGHTIES

Amal Shamma'*

While the focus of this conference is on the individual child who is battered by individual adults in isolated incidents, this paper will deal with the problem of mass brutalization of the children of a whole society by the organized activity of their society or of another, specifically the problem of children and war.

Over the last 40 years there have been many wars, almost all in the Third World. The countries concerned have witnessed the deaths of large numbers of their populations, the destruction of their natural resources, the undermining of their national institutions, the disruption of their planned development and targeted progress, and a diversion of already scarce national funds from social areas of need towards military expenditure.

The effect all this has had on the health, welfare, and development of the child is the subject of this discussion. Particular reference will be made to the decade-long war in Lebanon.

1. The Physical Effects: War is a Major Killer of Children

Wars affect children in many ways. Of the most obvious and dramatic are the immediate, physical effects.

War is a major killer of children in the Third World. In Lebanon, an estimated 120,000 people have died since 1975. A random review of the listings of the dead any day in the Lebanese press would put the proportion of children below 15 years at anywhere between 15% and 33%; in other words, 18,000 to 40,000 children have been killed by the war in Lebanon over 10 years. No single disease can boast the same killing rate in the same period of time.

In 1982, during the Israeli invasion of Lebanon, 19.3% of civilian casualty admissions to Berbir Medical Center in Beirut were below 15 years of age, and 11.4% of those died. These figures do not include those transferred to other centres or those who died in the emergency room before admission.

A crucial point to be made here is that war is not listed in public health classification manuals, national or international, as a cause of death of children. As a result, there is no established mechanism for the effective collection and reporting of pertinent statistical information relating to the subject. Sporadic, limited or anecdotal statistical analyses can never reveal the magnitude of the problem, as is evident from the Lebanese examples stated above.

Many children who do not die in a war are injured in it. In a review of admissions of paediatric war injuries to the Berbir Medical Center during the Israeli invasion of Lebanon in 1982, 82% of the cases were seen to have suffered moderate and severe injuries, with major handicaps occuring in 13.5%. Facilities for managing such handicaps in Lebanon are limited.

Children are also subject to political kidnapping and torture and several cases have been reported in Lebanon.

* Pediatrician, Barbir Hospital, Beirut, Lebanon

2. The Social and Economic Effects: War Denies Children their Rights

The social and economic effects of war on children are more subtle to discern, more difficult to measure, and, consequently, even less known to the public and policymakers than the physical effects of war.

War disrupts the economy of the country that stages it, interrupts development and progress, contributes to poverty, unemployment and inflation, destroys natural, human and established resources, increases despair, and decreases creative initiative.

Children in the war zone, when not targets of shelling, suffer from the death of parents and providers, and from homelessness, malnutrition, insufficient medical care, interrupted formal education and stunted personal growth.

In Lebanon thousands of children have been orphaned, tens of thousands of families do not live in their homes, agricultural regions have been devastated, major industrial areas have been destroyed, schools and hospitals have been either damaged or rendered non-operational, public services barely exist, and governmental strategies affecting health, education, housing, and economic growth have virtually halted.

The preparation for war in the Third World countries may be even more devastating to those countries' growth and well-being. Harfouche, in a review of the effect of increasing militarism in the world, describes the effects of an unprecedented competition between militarization and social development for those countries' already scant resources.

She shows that funds expended on the military, even in industrialized nations, far exceed what is spent on health research, energy resource development, and feeding and housing for the poor. In developing nations the imbalance is even greater, with spending on arms purchases far outstripping what is spent on health, education, sanitation, agriculture, etc. In addition, Third World countries can expect 20 times less in economic assistance from industrialized countries than the amount that these devote to their own military expenditure.

While military expenditures throughout the world continue to grow, global output has not kept up. At present, the poor, the malnourished, the illiterate in the world are in ever-increasing numbers, as are those who lack adequate housing, medical care, and safe environments.

Not only has the financing of the military brought neither peace nor security but also it is directly linked to the worsening economic and social conditions world-wide, which, in turn, increases the likelihood of war in the Third World.

3. The Psychological Effects: Children Brought up in War may Advocate War as Adults

The psychological effect of war on children has received some study, though far from adequate. In Lebanon several researchers, using various techniques, have investigated the psychological, social and moral effects of the war on Lebanese children.

Yacoub (1978) studied 30 children, and their families and paediatricians, and noted evidence of increased fearfulness, insecurity, regression in behaviour, sleep disturbances and nightmares, among those living in the war zone. Nassar (1985), in her study of children, noted problems in relating to others, insecurity, lack of self-esteem, poor self-image, depression, dependency, feelings of guilt, isolation, and a rigid super-ego.

What may be most significant are the long-term effects of prolonged exposure of children to war. Yacoub noted in some of his subjects a fascination with, and desire for participation in, the acts of killing.

Abu Nasr *et al.* (1978) studied 548 children aged 11 to 14 years to detect the effect of their exposure to war on their moral judgement. Results indicated that a full 26% of the children changed their judgement from a moral one to an immoral one with respect to the acceptability of killing, irrespective of their age, sex, religion, social class or extent of exposure to war.

A common scene on a paediatric ward where casualties are treated is to see the injured play with their favourite toys: toy machine-guns and toy soldiers. These same children may fantasize that their injuries were inflicted as they "butchered their enemies". Children wander into hospital grounds and help pick up pieces of bodies and carry the dead to the morgue. In their homes, children talk of gory scenes, massive injury, and death of neighbours, with remarkable detachment. The streets are usually the arena for the war-games of children emulating their heroes, the militia-men of the neighbourhood.

In a country where anywhere between 35% and 51% of the population is below the age of 15 years, a war lasting 10 years would mean that at least two thirds of the children have never known peace, have lived in isolated communities, and have grown up when violent people, the militia-men, were heroes. The children of 1975, ten years later, are the new militia-men of today, and killing has become their way of life.

For some children the transition from fantasy participation to real participation takes place much sooner. The phenomenon of child soldiers and militiamen has been seen in many Third World wars. Although, in some cases, children are actively recruited the more ominous are those instances where children insist on joining the fighting forces to participate in the war. Such is the case in Lebanon.

In addition, significant changes have occurred in social mores among Lebanese youth, ranging from an increased incidence of drug abuse to the appearance of child prostitution, to a return to religious fundamentalism, to an acceptance of non-traditional moral codes, to a disdain for the work ethic and the merit system, and to a retreat from national commitment to one of self-preservation.

4. A Plan of Action for Health Workers

The immensity of the problems of children in war dictate a many-faceted response that would involve the health worker at all levels of expertise and fields of action.

One of the most important and immediate objectives was delineated by Harfouche. She forcefully advanced the argument that war should be recognized to be the leading killer of children in the Third World, and preparation for war the leading deterrent to the advancement and accessibility of health for families and children.

She suggests that this hypothesis be tested and the adverse effects of war on families and children quantified and subsequently controlled by a mechanism which the Division of Family Health of the World Health Organization would establish. This should entail the development of an international record system reporting child deaths and injuries resulting from war operations, as is the case with other statistically classifiable causes of mortality and morbidity. She recommends a revision of the International Classification of Diseases (ICD) to include war operations and resulting injuries as a distinct category. She also recommends the use of lay or paramedical personnel for the reporting of data to facilitate application of the system in developing countries.

The impact of seeing war heading the list of causes of death of children constantly, in national and international documents, might help to bring home to policymakers in every country the need to control militarization to save their own children's lives.

Such a course of action should create an awareness among peoples and governments that disarmament and the prevention of war are imperative conditions not only for peace but also for the realization of the principles set forth in the Declaration of Human Rights and the Declaration of the Rights of the Child. The stated goal of achieving health for all by the year 2000 will not be attained if militarization and war continue at the present pace.

The health worker can also take the lead in efforts to halt the social and economic consequences of accelerating militarism in both developed and developing countries. Making known to policymakers and to the public what vast social, medical, environmental, educational, and nutritional accomplishments could be attained by the diversion of some of the ingenuity, research, technology, and funds away from military programmes might bring about a realization that greater peace and security could be achieved by addressing the needs of human societies rather than by seeking greater destructive capabilities.

It has been shown repeatedly that the diversion of just a small proportion of the funds used by the military could improve the possibility and the quality of life for millions of people in developed and developing countries. A mere 5% of those funds could eliminate hunger, control disease, and provide housing and productive employment for millions. Alternative priorities that could be funded by such a diversion of monies away from militarization have been listed, and these lists should continue to be brought to the attention of policymakers and the public in an effort to encourage such a course of action world-wide.

A final, important note to be made concerns the future of the Third World. War has the same effects as poverty, ignorance, disease and malnutrition in crippling a developing country and inhibiting the appearance within it of motivated, creative, capable individuals who can lead it towards its national goals of health, food, and education for all. Children brought up in war, made to view violence as acceptable behaviour in resolving problems, will be unlikely to shun violence as adults. In particular, killing may not always be regarded as immoral. On a national scale, their generation, when faced with regional disputes, could both opt for and support financing and engaging in war. The cycle of militarism leading to poverty, despair and further militarism would have been firmly established.

References

[1] Harfouche, J.K. *Intra-species War: a Major Killer of Children in the Third World; What Can We Do About It?* 1981.
[2] Harfouche, J.K. *Impact of Man-made Disasters on Family and Child Health* 1980.
[3] Yacoub, G., *Psychological Disturbances in Lebanese Children During and After the War.* Educational Council for Research and Development, 1978.

4 Nassar, C., *Psychological Effects of the War on Lebanese Children of Various Social Groups.* Doctoral Thesis, Sorbonne University, Paris, 1985.
5 Abu Nasr, J. *et al. Moral Judgement of Lebanese Children After the Lebanese War.* Institute for Women's Studies, Beirut University College, 1978.

SEXUAL ABUSE AND CHILD PROSTITUTION

Judith Ennew*

Since the 1970s there has been public concern about the sexual exploitation of children in the United States of America and in Europe. Commentators in both places seem to assume that there is an increased interest in sex for recreational rather than procreational purposes and that this leads to satiation and dissatisfaction with so-called normal forms of heterosexual activity and a consequent interest in other forms of stimulus, such as sex with children. This is frequently linked to a reported increase in prostitution and pornography. It has been suggested that powerful "industries" in child prostitution and pornography have developed, and terms like "baby pros" and "kiddie porn" have entered current use. Linked allegations suggest that an international traffic in children exists on a large scale and that "sex tours" are organized so that men from the developed world can visit exotic countries for erotic experiences with children. The issue has been well covered by both journalists and academics and is linked to current debates on sexual freedom, child rights, and feminism.

This apparent trend in the sexual exploitation of children has not been without official investigation (Government of Canada 1984; Boudhiba 1982; Fernand-Laurent 1983). Research is also being carried out by non-governmental organizations like the Odessy Institute in the United States, the National Society for the Prevention of Cruelty to Children in the United Kingdom, and the International Society of Abolitionists. Special units have been established to research the incidence, effects and prevention of sexual abuse of children and to develop modes of rehabilitation of victims.

Despite so much interest at so many levels, the picture is by no means clear and this is partly because many people find it difficult to deal with the notion of childhood sexuality or to separate work in this field from moral campaigns. To take one instance of confusion: there is no logical or proven progression from increased heterosexual activity to satiation, or yet from satiation to a search for abnormal sexual gratification. Indeed, if this were the case, sexually active marriages might also be regarded as responsible for increased prostitution and pornography. Similarly, there are no exact criteria for defining sexual precocity. Moreover, psychoanalysts have been debating hotly for 80 years whether children desire adults or are victims of adult desire. No accurate statistics are available for sexual abuse and exploitation, and the wildest 'guestimates' are often treated as official figures, while unsubstantiated anecdotes and journalism may be referred to as 'evidence' and 'research'. Thus the real situation is obscured by the repetition of poorly documented facts and speculation. Within the recent debate regarding child sexual abuse there is often a prurient element, which leads to sensational treatment. Meanwhile, such terms as "kiddie porn" and "baby pro" degrade childhood dignity, in the same way that women are degraded by being called "chicks" or "girls".

To avoid these problems it is necessary to examine child sexual abuse in the

* Cambridge Institute for the Study of Industrial Societies, Kings College, 30 Mill Lane, Linton, Cambridge CB1 6JY, England

context of the whole range of possible sexual relationships in which it occurs. This means looking at physical acts and biological facts and also at social structures of gender and power. Childhood sexuality is caught up in two sets of power relations: those between men and women and those between adults and minors. It is also necessarily entangled in economic power relations, because women and children are generally economically dependent on adult males. But class and race also play their part in sexual exploitation. A child's dependence and need for protection are not just a natural result of biologically determined innocence, but arise from pre-existing imbalances of power which render him or her vulnerable to all kinds of exploitation.

Although the definition of childhood has many historical and cross-cultural variations, some kind of status distinction between adult and non-adult societal members is universal in human societies and the distinction is made according to the presence or absence of secondary sexual characteristics. Infants and pre-pubertal children are visibly different from reproductively mature adults. It is post-pubertal "adolescents" who present definitional problems in many societies. Physically adult-sized and able to reproduce, they are nevertheless regarded as needing measures of protection or control for sexual and other purposes. Society requires them to undergo further socialization and education before they achieve adult status and they usually need to acquire the means of economic independence before they can assume the role of parent.

The key physiological factor is that in pre-pubertal individuals reproductive organs are undeveloped, or in the process of developing. But even the biological definition of "sex" cannot be entirely limited to visible reproductive features. Their development and functioning are dependent on the endocrine system, which affects the well-being of the whole person. Thus it is always incorrect to reduce "sex" to genital activity. Sexual abuse of children may include non-genital touching, threatening behaviour, adult exhibitionism or showing sexually explicit material to non-consenting children. One witness to a United States House of Representatives inquiry defined child sexual exploitation as "any act committed by an adult designed to stimulate a child sexually, or any act in which the child is used for the sexual stimulation of an adult" (Swift 1978).

Physical harm may not be a necessary outcome of intergenerational sexual activity. Much depends upon the child's age and physical development. Doctors have reported cases of small children suffering from poor sphincter control, anal and vaginal lacerations, and asphyxiation as a result of sexual contact with adults. Girls who have reached the menarche are at risk of pregnancy, which they may be unable to support physically, socially or economically. Sexually transmitted diseases may have particularly devastating consequences for immature individuals (Barry et al., 1984 p. 99; WHO in Fernand-Laurent, 1983, p. 32). However, case histories of Western children show that physiological damage is less noticeable than psychological harm. Many cases are discovered only because children exhibit a variety of psychosomatic symptoms or behavioural problems such as bed-wetting or aggressive behaviour (Vizard, 1984). In cases where neither physical harm nor psychological trauma result from what a child may have perceived as a warm and loving relationship, he or she can suffer damaging feelings of guilt because of the reactions of parents, police and doctors when the relationship is discovered. In other cases children may be emotionally harmed if they are rejected by an adult sexual partner once childhood is over and the adult no longer finds them attractive (Kraemer, 1976).

There are indications that some children are particularly vulnerable to adult sexual approaches because of parental rejection. As clinical research increases it is also becoming evident that many child abusers were themselves abused as children. It is therefore not surprising to note that, despite the widely accepted public image of the abuser as a threatening stranger, it can be argued from recent evidence that most sexual relationships between adults and children take place between members of the same family, household or social group. Evidence also suggests that this is not limited to Western societies.

The idea that sexual abuse is largely perpetrated by strangers persists partly because incest rules are some of the most fundamental of all social norms; breaches of them tend to arouse the strongest feelings of anger and abhorrence as well as the most extreme punishments. Families in which incestuous relationships exist keep their silence because of fear of social censure. Society as a whole would rather pretend that such relationships do not exist at all, or that they are rare abnormalities. It is a common belief in Western societies that incest rules are universal in form and based on biological imperatives: that reproductive behaviour between close biological kin results in the birth of deformed children. But this is not the case. Whatever the biological facts, many societies prohibit marriage or sexual intercourse between people who have no biological connection: as in the case of societies which forbid a girl to marry any of the men who passed through initiation rites at the same time as her father. Incest rules often serve to draw the boundary of social rather than biological relationships. A common example is that sexual activity between stepfather and stepdaughter is regarded as incestuous, despite the lack of blood relationship.

The most common recorded form of intergenerational incest is between fathers or stepfathers and daughters. But intrafamilial sexual activity is not always intergenerational. The British Incest Survivors Campaign has stated that 30% of the reports it receives concern assaults on sisters by brothers. It is also incorrect to assume that it is only female children who suffer abuse. Although the abuser is nearly always an adult or older male, victims are frequently boys or male adolescents.

The fact that most sexual abuse of children occurs with known adults has two consequences. First, it throws doubt upon some of the assumptions of moral crusaders who make use of material relating to child sexual exploitation. Such campaigns often relate an apparent increase in occurrence of sexual abuse to a breakdown of family values. They emphasize the image of the abuser as a stranger and also make much of the commercial sexual exploitation of children by means of prostitution and pornography. Exaggeration and distortion of these aspects obscure the problems within families and leave many children at risk of abuse. Second, the child suffers a confusion of loyalties and emotions. Paradoxically, parents who abuse their children often reveal an overvaluation of family values. It is not unusual to hear the claim that parental rights include sexual rights or that a parent is a particularly sensitive and acceptable sexual teacher. In the resultant confusion of loyalties and emotions the child sees the powerful parental figure as both provider and lover, even if society regards the action as abuse and even if the child has suffered physical damage.

Sexual abuse within the family, by known individuals, or even by threatening strangers, must be distinguished from exploitation of children's sexuality for profit by means of prostitution or pornography. The central fact which distinguishes prostitution from other forms of economic sexual institutions, like bride-price and concubinage, is that it involves a market transaction for a specific service. A price is set for a sexual act or acts. The negotiation involves a purchaser (client), a seller (prostitute or agent), and a commodity (sexuality). In the case of child prostitution, the purchaser and the agent are usually both adults, although it is not always the case that child prostitutes operate with the protection of pimps or procurers. But the clients are adults and thus child prostitutes are subjected to a double exploitation, of their sexuality and of their childhood.

A distinction must be drawn between pre-pubertal child prostitutes and post-pubertal minors who are involved in prostitution. It has been observed that there is a strong preference for young people among clients for both male and female prostitutes. This may be related to the spread of Western overvaluation of youthful characteristics, as well as to an association between youth, vigour and potency. Beauty is youth, rather than truth, in popular culture. Most available evidence about so-called child prostitutes refers not to pre-pubertal children but to young people who have not reached political majority. There *is* a market for young children, but I would suggest that it is not so large as moral crusaders would wish us to believe. Nor is it necessarily the basis for a profitable industry. Pre-pubertal child prostitutes may be part of both high- and low-price prostitution. Some clients seek gratification for a specialized taste for contact with individuals of either sex who lack secondary sexual characteristics like pubic hair. Paedophilic customers are specifically interested in sex with children, partly to recapture their own idyllic and narcissistic image of childhood, partly because children are not seen as threatening sexual partners, as would be the case with adults. They may be willing to pay a high price for this sexual contact and often have to do so because both demand and supply are low. Scarcity increases the value, but the market is limited because paedophilia is related to romantic ideas of love and childhood. Purchased, short-term sex is not the most gratifying form for paedophiles and they are more likely to seek a longer relationship with a child they know.

The other market for pre-pubertal sexuality is particularly cheap and arises because of the availability of children for both sexual and economic exploitation in certain contexts. Vagrant children, unprotected by family or known adults, live in quite large numbers in urban areas of the developing world. They are particularly vulnerable to adult exploitation and available for cheap sex, to customers who are not primarily paedophiles but who are simply seeking sexual gratification of any kind for the lowest possible outlay. These customers are not usually rich degenerates but poor, unemployed and possibly homeless men. Street children may be exploited by adults or older youths who act as procurers and provide the children with food, drugs, shelter and a fiction of adult protection. On the other hand, children may sell their own sexuality directly to casual customers, often for as little as a packet of sweets or a handful of cigarettes (Ennew 1986).

The key to this market is the economic and political powerlessness of children. Once outside a family context or state welfare control, they have no legitimate means of acquiring food or shelter. The same is true of teenage runaways in developed countries, who are better documented than Third World street-children. Studies of child prostitution in the United States and Europe suggest that many minors become prostitutes after leaving home and travelling hopefully to towns and cities, where they find themselves friendless, hungry and homeless. Because legislation bars them from legal employment, they may have no means of obtaining a living other than prostitution. Moreover, in the efficient bureaucracies of industrial societies it is difficult for them to evade police or welfare surveillance and avoid being either sent home or put into state care. Pimps and brothel-owners are adept at providing new documents with an adult identity. Threats of exposure or gratitude for the services rendered make these documents a means of inducing young runaways to sell their sexuality. However, contrary to popular ideas of such young people as sex slaves, case histories provided by researchers, like Gitta Sereny, seem to indicate that young prostitutes are not tied to particular adults and are able to change exploiters with relative ease. Nevertheless pimps do serve an important psychological function for many runaways, becoming father figures as well as lovers to girls who may have lacked parental affection. The situation of runaway boys is slightly different. The paternal model, allied to male dominance over females, allows pimps to intervene between clients and girl prostitutes. Boys tend to enter prostitution through a system of adult-male patronage. The man/boy relationship is not built on explicit exploitation but cast in the form of love or friendship. Clients for a girl's sexuality are more likely to be seeking quick, anonymous sexual release, while homosexual and heterosexual customers for boys may be seeking a relationship lasting anything from a few hours to several months, in which payment is more likely to be rendered in gifts and shelter than in money. The fact that boys do not work through intermediaries renders them more vulnerable to violence (Sereny 1984; Lloyd 1977).

Whilst many child prostitutes are runaway children, not all prostitutes are living outside a family group. Some children prostitute themselves in order to supplement pocket money on a casual basis. Some eventually run away, but many continue to live in relatively prosperous homes, having decided that their need for certain consumer items, such as clothes, records, tickets for discotheques, drugs or alcohol, is sufficient to make it worthwhile to sell their sexuality. They discover the market places of the consumer society as buyers and as sellers, the fault lying less with poor home conditions than with a culture which equates consuming with "feeling good". This type of casual prostitution is more likely to be prevalent in developed countries or among middle-class children, and is a result of relative wealth rather than relative poverty.

The market in young sexuality is often combined with the market in exotic sexuality. Modern tourism between Western and non-Western countries has emerged out of an exploitative system in which national images are manipulated for profit. Many host countries see tourism as the key to national growth, and a welcoming society may also be a prostituted society. A remark made by the then Deputy Prime Minister of Thailand in November 1980 has been widely quoted in this context:

> I ask all governors to consider the natural scenery in your provinces, together with some forms of entertainment that some of you might consider disgusting and shameful because they are forms of sexual entertainment that attracts tourists . . . ' (Perpignan, 1981, p. 543).

Some tourists travel in search of specifically sexual pleasures, seeking experiences which are prohibited in their own countries. For them, sexual entertainment, which may entail sexual relations with young partners, is the main purpose of the visit. Or they may be individuals who are inhibited from trying certain sexual options within their own cultures and seek exotic experiences which they may mistakenly believe to be "natural" to the host culture. For these customers sexual entertainment may be an ideal part of their more legitimate tourist activities; young or child partners are not specifically sought but might be tried experimentally. A further type of client in this range is not a tourist but a male visitor to another culture, who is separated from his usual sexual outlets or constraints. Japanese business men on overseas trips in South-East Asia are reported to be regular customers for sexual services. Men who work away from home in an all-male environment, such as sailors, military personnel and oil workers, are an important part of this category and it is not unusual for their employers to provide sexual entertainment for relaxation purposes. This is, of course, related to notions of male sexuality which assume that even quite short periods of celibacy are harmful. Some of the evidence relating to these cases shows that these customers do request very young prostitutes.

Whatever form it takes, "sex tourism" does not always or exclusively involve minors. Where it does, it exemplifies the way in which forms of domination can be interrelated. In "sex tourism" youth submits to age and female to male, while the inequality between inhabitants of rich and poor nations is combined with national class differentials, and the whole is complicated further by racial and ethnic discrimination. The two poles of the nexus are represented by rich, white, adult, Western males and poor, non-white, young, non-Western females.

Also, the use of children in pornography is an expression, not of social abnormality, but of the entire range of socio-sexual relationships. It involves the representation of sex or sexuality for the sole purpose of stimulating the consumer. It is thus distinguished from erotica by the decontextualization of sexual behaviour. Pornography trivializes sexual relationships by separating them from social life and establishing an imbalanced power relationship between the portrayed sexual object and the consumer. Although childhood sexuality is often portrayed in literature, it is visual pornography (using photographs, films or videos) which arouses concern, because it depicts real children taking part in sexual activities with each other or with adults for the stimulation of adult viewers (Tyler 1982). There is no necessary connection between pornography and material gain, for the representations are often produced for private or restricted use, perhaps in the course of a paedophilic relationship. Because they are amateur, they are often of poor quality, and it is a measure of the relatively restricted range of both supply and demand that poor-quality goods are frequently marketed. Most child pornography simply depicts children in varying degrees of nakedness and some of this is scarcely distinguishable from family snapshots. Such material is sold at anything from double to ten times the price of adult, heterosexual pornography, according to the country in which it is marketed. It is easily obtained in shops or by mail order. Pornography showing acts of intergenerational sexual intercourse is expensive, but the market is limited and the goods are comparatively difficult to obtain. Once again there are wide variations according to national legislations and tastes. What varies little is the product. A limited range of depictions appears repeatedly in the material sold under different labels. If there has been an increase in child pornography it is more likely to be due to advances in technology than to changing tastes. Photography changed the pornographic mode from depicting imaged acts to showing real events. Video and "instant" films have made it possible for amateurs and professionals to evade detection and prosecution. The child pornography which is found on national and international markets has its source in both amateur and professional circles and it is by no means clear that there is a vast profitable "kiddie porn" industry (Tyler, 1982; Schultz, 1980; Gersen, 1979).

Attempts have been made by various projects to tackle the problem of caring for young victims of sexual exploitation. One of the problems is that little is known about the incidence, effects and causes. Another is that what is known is often obscured by the prejudices of ideological crusades, whether these are religious, moral, feminist or liberationist. The Government of Canada has recently produced a report from which it is clear that one of the priorities for prevention is the education of both adults and children. This is echoed by several experimental projects in Europe and North America which treat victims, often together with their families, by educational initiatives which encourage children to speak out about child abuse and to learn how to say 'no' to adults. The crucial feature of all these programmes is the need to break the silence about sexual abuse by people related or known to the child, at the same time as increasing children's rights in society.

In the case of young prostitutes, rehabilitation is more difficult because they have been socialized into street life and criminal pursuits. Some are involved with drug consumption or dealing, others with petty theft and alcohol abuse. Street life, theft and prostitution all involve a life-style based on short-term gains: rapid cash return for minimum effort, combined with speedy spending on non-durable consumer goods. Rehabilitation schemes have to aim at educating minors to accept the delayed gratification which mature relationships, education and legitimate employment entail.

Rehabilitation schemes are by definition palliative. The aim should be to prevent the problem beginning. Harsher sanctions can be applied to offenders, but there is no evidence that these act as a deterrent. Many abusers have been shown to be victims themselves, and for those who pursue a life of hedonistic decadence prohibition may even make the act more attractive. Re-education rather than punishment might be a more suitable reaction to offences, particularly when the act involves a family group. Preventive work also needs to be oriented towards education and this should take place at three levels in society. First, children need to be taught how to recognize, avoid and reject sexual abuse. This can be done sensitively without injecting fear or disgust into the child's world view. Many interesting projects have developed in response to the recognition of the problem, using innovative methods. These may use dolls with explicit sexual features, which can be of particular use with younger children who lack a sophisticated vocabulary, or drama techniques in which ways of rejecting unwelcome approaches can be explored. At a second level, adults need to recognize the widespread incidence of incestuous abuse and to temper their reactions with a rational approach. Adults who have themselves been abused as children need sympathetic education about their own problems. All adults who deal with children as parents, professionals and friends need to be aware of the problems of child abuse, of the developmental needs of children, and also of the right of children to be respected socially and sexually. The third level of education relates to the societal reaction to sexual abuse of children, particularly the tendency to exaggerate and to use incorrect information as the basis of moral or political campaigns. What is needed is responsible and thorough research into all aspects of the sexual abuse of children.

References

Barry, K., Bunch, C. and Castley, S. (eds.) 1984 *International Feminism: Working against Female Sexual Slavery.* Report of the Global Feminist Workshop to Organise Against Traffic in Women, Rotterdam, Netherlands, April 6–15, 1983, International Women's Centre, New York.

Boudhiba, A. 1982 *Exploitation of Child Labour.* Final report of the Special Rapporteur of the Sub-Commission on Prevention of Discrimination and Protection of Minorities.

Ennew, J. 1986 (forthcoming) *The Sexual Exploitation of Children.* Polity Press.

Fernand-Laurent, J. 1983 Report of the Special Rapporteur on the Suppression of the Traffic in Persons and the Exploitation of the Prostitution of Others. United Nations Economic and Social Council, 17th March 1983; UN Geneva.

Gersen, R.L. 1979 *The Hidden Victims: the Sexual Abuse of Children,* Beacon Press, Boston, USA.

Government of Canada 1984 Summary of Sexual Offences against Children in Canada. Report of the Committee on Sexual Offences against Children and Youths: appointed by the Minister of Justice and Attorney General of Canada, and the Minister of National Health and Welfare.

Kraemer, W. (ed.) 1976 *The Forbidden Love: The Normal and Abnormal Love of Children,* Sheldon Press.

Perpignan, Sr. M.S. 1981 Prostitution Tourism. In: World Council of Churches, *Women in a Changing World,* No 11, Prostitution and Tourism.

Schultz, L.D. (ed.) 1980 *The Sexual Victimology of Youth.* Charles C Thomas, Springfield, Illinois, USA.

Sereny, G. 1984 *The Invisible Children: A Study of Child Prostitution,* André Deutch.

Swift, C. 1978 Sexual Assault of Children and Adolescents. Testimony to the House of Representatives, USA, 11th January 1978.

Tyler, T. 1982 *Child Pornography: the International Exploitation of Children.* Paper presented to the 4th International Congress on Child Abuse and Neglect.

Vizard, E. 1984 The Sexual Abuse of Children — Parts 1 & 2. *Health Visitor,* No. 157.

DISCUSSION

Lesnik Oberstein: I would like to raise a point with Dr Bell. I think that perhaps there is some more evidence for the role of adult psychopathology in child abuse than you seem to believe. Take child murder, for example, which we all agree is a form of child abuse. In a very thorough study by d'Orban in the British Journal of Psychiatry, in 1979, he reported on 89 mothers who had committed child murder and their families. He subdivided the mothers into six groups — the two largest groups he called "battering mothers" and "psychiatrically disturbed mothers". About 30 mothers were "battering", and about 20 were "psychiatrically disturbed". The "battering mothers" committed murder in response to provocation from the child. The psychiatrically disturbed mothers' murders were expressions of their illness. Now, this would seem to indicate that adult psychopathology may play a greater role.

Bell: My intention going through the models was to give a sort of historical account of their development. I did not preclude the fact that psychopathological factors could be included, although I do admit that perhaps in the paper I am less in favour of this psychopathological model. My concern is that, more often than not, people can often pick on psychopathology as being the prime cause, and I wanted to move our attention away from it, perhaps to a more interactionist analysis. It is certainly the case that the media tend to pick on that aspect of the problem.

Lesnik Oberstein: It seems to me that you were making the point, Mr. Reyes, that in non-industrialized countries it is a sociological factor, urbanization, that leads to child abuse; it then takes the specific form of child abandonment. If I understand you correctly, it seems to me very important that we in the industrialized countries become aware that our child-abuse models are not necessarily applicable to non-industrialized countries.

Reyes Romero: The policy in Colombia is to concentrate efforts in big cities, where all the children are together and there are more possibilities of abandoning children, as you say. So, I agree with you.

Ghobrial: I am a child psychiatrist from Egypt, in charge of the psychiatric clinic for schoolchildren in Cairo. In my experience over about 20 years I have found that the cause of the conditions for which most of the cases attended the clinics, such as speech difficulty, school retardation, behavioural disorders, school refusal, running away from school, lying, stealing, aggression, nervousness, obstinacy, on investigating them with the psychiatric social workers and the psychologists, was the maltreatment of the child at school and at home. At home, especially the mother, who is responsible for looking after her child in doing homework, treats him harshly because either he is slow or he does not understand well; at school the teachers beat him severely. Thus the child becomes a victim of both school and home. At the end the child is referred to the child psychiatry clinic for treatment for school retardation or some other problem. There, we use three approaches — psychotherapy for the child, parent guidance about how to treat the child and manage his homework, and contacting the child's teachers or the head of the school to advise them on how to treat him correctly. And lastly, we give lectures in schools. This is my role in helping the child who is abused.

Rapoport: My question to Dr. Reyes, who referred to Latin America as a whole, with no mention of Cuba, is whether he would say a few words about the comparison of Cuba with other Latin-American countries.

Reyes Romero: There are no vagrant children in Cuba because the social organization of the country is different and the ideology of the government is also different. The typical vagrant child is not seen in Cuba.

Owen: I am a lawyer from Britain working in health issues. My questions are directed to Dr Naidu and Dr Reyes. Can they help us with some answers about whether the law has any role to play in developing countries in relation to what they have been describing, such as abandoned children and child labour? I am totally confounded, particularly as regards India, by the enormous "explosion" of legislation. Some of this legislation is to ratify or to comply with International Labour Office standards and Conventions. Of course, a lot of the legislation in India is inherited from colonial statutes and is like other Commonwealth legislation. It is not always relevant to developing countries' actual circumstances. Equally, in Latin America many countries have ambitious family codes and labour laws which are well-intentioned but quite unrealistic. My question is this: a) should we be thinking about coming away from these somewhat unrealistic standards, because they are much too high, and instead try to find ways in which the law can be simplified and made more enforceable? For instance, in relation to child labour, we have to realize that children in these countries are working because that is the only way they can survive. Would it not be better to concentrate on ensuring that children who are working do not work in conditions that are dangerous to health and development? In particular, should we be thinking about how to narrow the gap between school-leaving and employment, developing legislation to provide relevant vocational training; that is, presenting concrete alternatives to illegal or unacceptable activities?

Naidu: You have raised a point to which a whole day could be devoted in discussion. We have recently had several debates on revision of legislation with regard to child labour, particularly in India, and still the debate is on. The question is whether we can take an extreme position by introducing legislation to abolish child labour or ban it particularly in hazardous industries or occupations. The question is — what minimum legislation could our country implement which would have direct and indirect relevance to child labour? One answer which we are now emphasizing, is that we have to think what legal minimum age of entry into employment for children has to be set and implemented. If we say 14 or 15 or 12 or 13 years, it doesn't help. So keeping in mind today's reality, but also the final goal, that in, say, two decades, or whatever time one can stipulate, over a period of time, we would take certain other steps which would lead to the reduction of child labour and finally to its abolition. To that extent legislation can help if we can implement it. The second point is that we have to see the legislation in terms of other areas, education for instance, as you have pointed out. There we have a goal: constitutionally we are committed to universal primary education. But this is not happening. However, can we submit people who are not sending their children to school to any legislative punishment? We can't do that. So, for the time being, what we have to do is to take up at least those areas in which it is absolutely hazardous for the child to work, and to see that children don't work in them. We have had a three-day seminar recently on legislation on child labour and we are thinking of revising it. What the spirit of this is that we cannot stop child labour, that it is harsh reality and let's accept it. That will be another way to legitimize child labour. We have to accept the reality that children have to work, but we can lay down conditions and specify hours and minimum age of entry into employment in a given country.

Reyes Romero: Although in Colombia there is a project in the Congress for elaborating a code for minors, for young people, most of these marginal populations, unfortunately, even though there are judges for the purpose, are unable to get this service from the community; they cannot be protected by the judge.

Obikeze: My comment goes to Dr. Shamma'. It has to do with one of her propositions. Specifically she mentioned that it would appear that children who grew up in conditions of war would be likely — in the long run, when they have grown up — to have a high disposition to solving problems by means of war or violence rather than peace. I wonder whether this proposition has been tested or it is just a suggestion. I have the feeling that it is more or less a carry-over from probably what was found during the Second and First World Wars. I doubt whether this would apply in all cases. We have had a civil war in Nigeria, in 1967–1970, and the children who lived through this period, some of them in truly traumatic conditions, are now going through secondary school. The first set of them is at university and I don't seem to find that this proposition holds, namely that this cohort of children is more prone to violence than any other group of those who were not so exposed. So I wonder whether this has been tested.

Shamma': A study has been carried out in Lebanon by the psychology department of one of the local colleges, at two different periods during the Lebanese War, one after the first two years of the war and the second more recently. At both times the study indicated a change in the moral judgement of children who had lived through war, irrespective of their personal exposure to its effects. In the first study, about 570 children between the ages of 11 and 14 were examined. This age group was chosen because it was considered to be the age at which moral values were being established for the rest of the individual's life. There were no previous studies before the war to compare this with so what they did was to take these children and expose them to two different situations — one in which killing took place under so-called natural circumstances and another in which killing took place during a war situation. And at least one quarter of the children who had been so examined revealed a change in their moral acceptability of the killing, from one where killing to them was immoral under the so-called natural setting to one where it was acceptable during the war situation. This is as objective as it can be. The question as to whether or not any further studies have been done — there haven't been any further studies other than that one and then a subsequent study by the same group, which has reiterated the same findings as to the moral issues, moral effects of the war. These children have been taken from different backgrounds, different ages, different religious groups, different classes and different amounts of exposure to war, whether they have just heard about it, happen to live in the country, or whether they had actually been in a situation where somebody from the family had been injured or was fighting. And what was found, irrespective of their exposure to war, was that the rate of change of moral judgement about the killing, was the same. One of the things I want to say again, something you see very objectively, and that is you do see enough children who will participate actively in war for various reasons. I have interviewed a number of them. Very few will do it for ideological reasons: most of them will do it because they want to shoot a gun and a rifle and they want to participate. The other thing is that you do have children who are very interested in death and dying, and that is the most horrific aspect of all of this. I feel that sometimes I am more horrified by the killing than the children are and that they can tolerate it much more than I can.

Bettex: I would like to ask Dr. Shamma' something. It is approximately what you have told us just now. In your paper you mention very briefly the official militarization of children. We read in the press that children are used as soldiers or guerrillas. Could you comment on that?

Shamma': In some cases there is active induction of children into various fighting groups but in most cases that I know of, particular to Lebanon, the children who have taken up arms and gone to the front — which doesn't have to be anything more than their neighbourhood street — have done so at their own insistence, not at any prodding by adults. They have done so because they have wanted to do so. Most of the children I have seen and talked to who carry arms have done so because they have wanted to.

Goodwin: I would ask anyone on the panel who would care to comment, but particularly Drs Bell and Ennew, whether they feel — and I am not sure to what extent this is a British phenomenon or whether it extends outside of Britain — the availability of home videos to young children, particularly those which contain very violent scenes of war, sexual violence, murder, and so on, is likely to lead to the same sort of change in moral values to which other speakers have referred?

Bell: I am not an expert in this particular area of violence on film or television and its effects on children, although I have noticed that there are large differences between individual countries, and it does seem that "video nasties", as they are called in the UK, are much more prevalent in England than in some other countries and more immediately available. Perhaps this is linked with economic conditions. At any rate, video-recording as a sort of activity carried out in the home seems to be quite prevalent in the United Kingdom, and I think it is possibly following a trend set in the United States.

Ennew: The whole business of video in the UK is quite interesting — we have got more videos per head of population than any other country. The point I would make in response to your question has to do with the general availability of new techniques like video and "instant" film and the effect this has had on the development of pornographic materials in general. It is much easier to make them without detection now. You can make your own videos, your own pornography videos, and show them to yourself, and an awful lot is made for private rather than commercial use, and the same goes for "instant" films. The violence aspect is often tied in with the pornography, particularly when it comes to children — and I am not talking about the exposure of children to it necessarily at this point, but sexual exploitation of children has to do with the power relations between adults and children, and therefore it is often shown in violent forms — the ultimate form being a "snuff movie", where children are actually killed in the course of the movie or video, or it is shown to be — apparently they are killed, and of course this happens with women as well, and this is an expression of male dominance over women.

SOCIAL POLICY AND SERVICE
ASPECTS OF THE PROBLEM

CHILD ABUSE AND NEGLECT: LEGAL AND JURIDICAL ASPECTS

Margaret Owen*

Child abuse and neglect have always been with us, throughout all our history, permeating our various diverse cultures. In the past it seems that societies did not seem too much concerned about it. A reading of some of the great English nineteenth century classics, such as Oliver Twist, Jane Eyre, Tom Brown's Schooldays, and The Water Babies, gives graphic indications of how children were viewed and treated a hundred years ago. Exploitation of the child within and outside the family was commonplace; abuse and neglect occurred in the factories, the workhouse, the public school and the nursery. Baby-farming killed off many an unwanted love-child; yet cruelty to animals was made a criminal offence a good 60 years before the equivalent treatment of children. The sponsor of the English 1889 child protection legislation was "anxious that we should give children *almost* the same protection as we give . . . domestic animals[1]." In New York in 1873 an eight-year-old child was removed from persons to whom she had been indentured, by the Society for the Prevention of Cruelty to Animals, on the ground that being a member of the animal kingdom her case fell within the animal cruelty laws[2]. The prosecution of the girl's mistress in 1874 led to the founding of the New York Society for the Prevention of Cruelty to Children.

Today, in developed countries, institutionalized abuse of the minor outside the family has almost disappeared through the enforcement of stringent laws on child labour, education and training, and entertainment, and the development of relatively effective monitoring mechanisms to ensure the child's protection in the public arena. Alarmingly, however, the reported incidence of intra-familial abuse and neglect has soared to quite epidemic proportions: in Canada, the United States of America, West Germany, and Britain, child sexual abuse is increasingly reported, within and outside the family. This September the United Kingdom National Society for the Prevention of Cruelty to Children (NSPCC) published its annual child abuse figures: the number of reported cases of physical abuse of children under 15 has risen by 70% in six years — with the biggest individual rise for reported cases of sexual abuse. Almost every week in Britain, harrowing stories of murder and abuse of children fill the newspapers, and public enquiries follow with tragic repetition.

These "reported" cases are only the tip of the iceberg. Many so-called "non-accidental injuries" never come to the notice of courts because of the difficulties of legal proof, and this inhibits the intervention of social services and child-care agencies. Emotional abuse is inevitably more hidden, difficult to define and identify, but it can result in the permanent damage of a child's personality and potential to develop into a capable and fulfilled adult.

In developing countries, aspects of extrafamilial abuse and neglect are well-known but responses to it are difficult to develop and implement. We know about debt-bondage, child-slavery, exploitation in factories and in home-based production; "forced" marriages; female circumcision; abduction, kidnap and

---

* Barrister-at-Law, 1, Horbury Crescent, London W.113.N.F., England

sale; child prostitution; exploitation of children for pornography; degrading ritual treatment; use of children for begging. All these practices have been the subject of many reports and research as well as international conventions and laws. The International Year of the Child revealed much about child maltreatment hitherto hidden from the limelight. Of intrafamilial abuse less has been revealed, for what goes on within the private realm of the family is obviously more difficult to report. It may be that traditional societies with the extended family protect the child from the horrific family abuse known in the West; however, this phenomenon is beginning to be detected there also, among families uprooted, through migration and poverty, from their traditional settings and age-old customs. But with poor resources, without a sophisticated network of social services, child care, education, welfare, or police surveillance, the child of impoverished parents in the barrios and shanty towns of Third World cities is inevitably vulnerable to maltreatment. The plight of the street children of Colombia, Mexico and Brazil has often been documented. Child prostitutes, as young as nine, kidnapped in Nepal to work in Bombay brothels, are at last attracting international concern.

The quality of children's lives on, for example, plantations demands urgent attention. As for neglect, it takes many forms. It can range from extreme ends of the spectrum, such as failure to feed or to feed adequately, resulting in malnutrition, to coldness, rejection, verbal abuse, and educational deprivation. Neglect of the child can be as traumatic as physical abuse but more difficult to detect.

The literature on child abuse and neglect world-wide is now considerable; but, although in the West juridical and legal aspects of the problem have been studied closely, the material coming from developing countries has concentrated in the main on the sociocultural factors contributing to child maltreatment. Implementation of child-protection legislation, the procedures for identifying, reporting, punishing the offender, and rehabilitating the child, and the actual administrative, legal, and judicial procedures have not been subjected to adequate scrutiny. A review of the juridical and legal aspects on child abuse in developing countries must be regarded as a priority research area.

To keep the subject within manageable limits, the main focus of attention in this paper will be on intrafamilial abuse. Although some reference will be made to the legislative texts in a few developing countries, the author has not been able to obtain information about the procedures for enforcing these laws, so juridical approaches considered will be mostly from Western countries, in particular, Britain. Some of these approaches are theoretically available in some developing countries, in the Commonwealth for instance, or might be adapted to other jurisdictions.

Nevertheless, there are certain commonalities between developed and developing countries, underscoring the intervention of the lawyer and the courts in the process of protecting the child against abuse and neglect. Parents have rights, often protected under the constitution, or family codes or at common law; children also have rights, and each have certain duties and obligations to each other. It is the balance between these two co-existing rights and those of the State that challenges the lawyer, child welfare agencies, the police and the judiciary.

The child's right to be protected against ill-treatment and abuse, and to have proper care, education and upbringing, countervails the parents' rights to decide the method of child-rearing, including correction and disciplining. In some countries, particularly those where there are greater resources to support child-caring agencies, education and health services, the law's intrusion into the private relationship of parent and child may be greater than in those which, while in no way condoning child abuse or neglect inside or outside the family, have not adequate facilities.

Courts generally respond to individual incidents of violence by identifying their legal components and invoking either the penal provisions of the criminal law or the compensatory machinery of civil litigation. But where intrafamilial abuse takes place, there may be sound reasons, such as the rehabilitation of the family, for not invoking the criminal law, while for the civil child-protection laws to be effective someone must initiate the procedure by alerting the welfare authorities to the fact that a child is or may be abused. In developing countries this obligation usually devolves upon the police; in developed countries other individuals and agencies may start investigations, such as social and health workers, doctors, teachers and voluntary organizations. The recurrent problem with most child protection legislation is that laws are unrealistic and ineffective. Clearly and urgently, the child, being the most vulnerable and least articulate member of society, merits special representation and some national "watchdog" authority, so that better legislation protects the minor in practice as well as in theory.

LEGAL DEFINITIONS

There can be no universally accepted definition of child abuse. As Kempe (1973)[3] explains "child abuse is not what the doctor thinks it should be; nor what the social worker thinks it is; but actually what the Courts say it is". Yet definition is the very essence of the law: without a clear definition the law is useless. Laws can' define abuse so broadly that its meaning is too ambiguous for the law to intervene; or so narrowly that many acts which constitute neglect and maltreatment escape the law's coverage. Much depends on who is doing the defining and for what purpose. For example, a definition for 'management guidance, as for inclusion in at-risk registers in the United Kingdom, will be different from that used for the purpose of operational research or a reporting law (as in the United States of America). Doctors will use one definition and social workers and teachers another. Definitions of child abuse reflect ideological differences, cultural attitudes to childhood, punishment (corporal punishment), child-rearing, training. Even within one country it will be difficult for all involved professionals to agree on what actually constitutes "neglect". The definition of "emotional abuse" is even more difficult. The definition used by the United Kingdom's National Society for the Prevention of Cruelty to Children (NSPCC) is helpful as a starter to this discussion: "All physically injured children under the age of 16 where the nature of the injury is not consistent with the account of how it occurred or where other factors indicate that there is a reasonable suspicion that the injury was inflicted or not prevented by any person having custody of the child." This is a fairly narrow definition, and ignores emotional damages. The United States has proposed an amendment[4] to Article 8 of the Draft Convention on the Rights of the Child " . . . all forms of physical or mental injury or abuse, general neglect or negligent treatment, sexual abuse or exploitation, or maltreatment caused by the child's parent(s), legal guardian(s), or any other person responsible for the child's welfare under circumstances which indicate that the child's welfare is harmed or threatened." A reference such as this, in a statute, to "sexual abuse" might assist in its detection and prevention.

Any definition selected may have important implications for civil liberties, that is, the conflicting rights, described above, of parents, children and the State, as it may also have for the allocation of scarce resources. Lawyers are likely to define child abuse differently from doctors and social workers, and may be prepared to intervene only in the most serious cases, where all the elements in the definition can be proved either on the criminal or on the civil standard of proof. Teachers, doctors, social workers and voluntary agencies may be anxious to intrude wherever there is any risk to the child immediately or in the foreseeable future. But the child needs protection before the injury occurs: prevention is more important than punishment of the offender after the event.

Under the English *Children's and Young People's Act, 1969* the grounds for proceeding for a care order are:

   a)   the child's proper development is being avoidably prevented or neglected or his health is being avoidably impaired or neglected or he is being ill-treated; or

   b)   this is or has been the case with regard to another child who is or was in the same household or a person who is or who may become part of the child's household was convicted of an offence against the child; or

(c,d,e,f) that the child is exposed to moral danger or beyond the control of his parent or guardian or is not receiving full-time education or is guilty of any offence (this last category is rare); *and* that he is in need of care or control which he is unlikely to receive unless the court makes an order. (sections 1 and 2). In addition, the *Child Care Act, 1980,* broadly re-enacting earlier legislation provides, under section 2, that a child under 17 shall be received into care (i.e. not taken into care against the parents' wishes) if he is abandoned or an orphan, or his parents are temporarily or permanently prevented from properly caring for him by reason of mental, physical, or other capacity or circumstances, and that the intervention of the local authority under the section is necessary for his welfare. In some situations the local authority can assume parental rights and these conditions are broader than under the 1969 Act — for example, if the child has been in voluntary care for three years; or the parent is unfit to have the care of the child by reason of permanent incapacity, mental disorder, habits or modes of life (e.g. vagrancy, drug addiction), or consistent failure to discharge the obligations of a parent. The conditions for assumption of parental rights under the Child Care Act of 1980 are substantially wider than those pertaining under the 1969 Act. The definitions, however, in both acts are undeniably broad, and it is up to the local authority to prove, on the balance of probabilities (the civil standard of proof), that the conditions exist. What the local authority may consider "impairs the proper development", what the doctor at the casualty department of the hospital regards as "ill-treatment" or what the social worker regards as "neglect" may still not satisfy the court. The court may interpret the definitions to meet what it regards as the legislator's true intention, while taking due note that any action by the State to take away parental rights has implications for civil liberties. For example, the removal of a child from the care of the parents infringes the child's right to family life and may prevent essential "bonding" with the mother.

Lawyers are likely to consider closely the abuser's mental state to see what his intentions really were, and whether the act was committed deliberately or recklessly. Professionals in the caring services may feel that the mental state of the perpetrator of the act (or omission) is of less significance than the fact that the injury resulted from an accident whilst the child was in his or her care.

Accidents pose a problem to the would-be definer of child abuse. It is not always easy to distinguish intentional from accidental behaviour. A series of accidents may persuade a court that the person taking care of the victim has been at least negligent in not taking greater care. In an American case[5] a one-year-old child was admitted to hospital after swallowing some bleach from a bottle left on the kitchen floor. The child was discharged after treatment and the parents warned to take greater care. A month later the child was again hospitalized in the same circumstances and the doctor filed a "neglect" report. The court found that "the distinction between accidental and non-accidental injury has no significance with regard to a child's safety when the accident is part of a pattern of neglect." A legal definition might accommodate such a conclusion.

The dangers inherent in developing narrow and precise definitions of child abuse become apparent when the cultural content of child abuse is recognized. Thus, the child-rearing patterns of an identifiable minority, who are either much stricter or more permissive than the prevailing population, may lead to insensitive and misguided judicial interventions. Similarly, families who, through no fault of their own, live in relative or absolute poverty may of necessity deny to their children what the wider establishment (and better-off community) regard as the minimum resources of childhood: own room, holidays, excursions, toys, a varied diet. Intervention, in this situation, may more easily take the shape of removing the child from its family rather than reallocating resources to alleviate the effects of poverty, thus keeping the home intact.

Invariably, in most of the legislation in operation around the world, there is reference to the danger to the child's "moral welfare". However, use of this expression is yet another example of how definitions of child abuse can drift into vagueness and subjectivity. Tests of morality in Western and Westernized countries tend to centre upon sexual activity; the exposure of young girls to the risk of pregnancy, abortion, and sexually-transmitted diseases provides some justification for this approach. But intervention in the parent-child relationship via judicial order may be inappropriate: the condition of the child may not be due to any act or omission of the parent, and the use of a definition which is incident-oriented may result in grave injustices.

Statutory tests of abuse and neglect in some selected countries

An analysis of the various statutory tests of a "neglected" child or a "child in need of protection" reveals an exceptionally broad range of criteria for state intervention[6]. In Canada alone, Roman Komar found 38 diverse definitions (demonstrating the breadth, subjectivity, cultural and aesthetic components of child maltreatment) in the different jurisdictions, and many dramatic contrasts between them. For example, of the 38 categories, Ontario's laws covered 11, Quebec's 6, and Newfoundland's 24. In Sweden since 1980 drug abuse is a ground for a care order.

A number of countries with civil law jurisdictions base their child protection legislation on the old Roman Law notion of *patria potestas*. The rights, duties, and obligations of parenthood are spelt out either broadly or in more detail, and it is the breach of these duties which provides the State with the power to deprive one or both parents of *patria potestas* or suspend their exercise of it. In these systems, the legal definitions of child abuse and neglect tend to be parent- or guardian-related, rather than focused on the conditions of the child.

The Cuban Family Code of 1975 is a good example of this type of definition. Article 85 spells out the rights and duties of the parents as follows:

(i) Keeping their children under their guardianship and care; making every possible effort to provide them with a *stable home and adequate nourishment;* caring for their *health and personal hygiene;* providing them with the means of recreation fitting their age which are within their possibilities; giving them the *proper protection;* seeing to their good behaviour and cooperating with the authorities in order to overcome any situation or environmental factor that may have an unfavourable effect on their training and development.

(ii) Seeing to the education of their children; inculcating them with the love for learning; seeing to it that they attend school; seeing to their adequate technical, scientific and cultural improvement in keeping with their aptitude and vocation and the demands posed by the country's development; and collaborating with the educational authorities in school programmes and activities.

(iii) Training their children to be useful citizens; inculcating them with the love of their country, respect for the country's symbols and their country's values, the spirit of internationalism, the standards of co-existence, and socialist morality; respect for social property and the property and personal rights of others; arousing the respect of their children by their attitude towards them; and teaching them to respect the authorities, their teachers and every other person.

(iv) Administering and caring for their children's property; seeing to it that their children use and enjoy in a proper manner whatever property they have; and not to sell, exchange or give any such property except in the interest of the children and pursuant to the requisites of this Code.

Article 86 specifically empowers the parent to discipline the child: "The parents are invested with the authority to reprimand and set straight adequately and moderately those children under their *patria potestas*". There seems little possibility of defining corporal punishment as a type of "abuse" in Cuba and similar civil law jurisdictions. Note how in this legislation the State has introduced a political aspect of child-rearing into the definition: parents who may question "respect for the country's values" may find that their *patria potestas* is challenged in the courts, and their conduct classified as "neglect". Article 95 goes on to add that where one or both parents:

1) are grossly derelict in their duties as established in Article 85;
2) induce the child to carry out a criminal act;
3) abandon the national territory and, therefore, their children;
4) observe a defective, corrupting, criminal or dangerous conduct incompatible with the exercise of *patria potestas*;
5) commit a crime against the child;

the court may remove or suspend *patria potestas*, and decide the childrens' future.

The Brazilian Civil Code (Art. 392) has similar provisions. By contrast with the Cuban Code, *patria potestas* can be removed if a parent inflicts "immoderate punishment". The Penal Code treats "maternal, intellectual and moral abandonment" as indictable crimes.

The Philippines Civil Law Code, Republic Act No. 386, 1975, Art. 356 enunciates the rights of every child to

a) parental care,
b) elementary education,
c) moral and civic training, and
d) physical, moral and intellectual training.

It goes on in some more detail to describe the rights: for example, the right to a balanced diet, adequate clothing, sufficient shelter, proper medical attention, and all the basic requirements of a healthy and vigorous life. Also[8] "the right to protection against exploitation, improper influences, hazards and other conditions or circumstances prejudicial to his physical, mental, emotional, social and moral development". Under the Civil Code, every child has the right to the "care and protection of the State, particularly when his parents or guardians fail or are unable to provide him with his fundamental needs for growth, development and improvement". This article has been construed as meaning that a child's rights are not dependent on the whims and caprices of the parents, and the State has a right to intervene where the upbringing is not in line with government policies and standards. The general feature of such codes is for child abuse to be defined not in a positive sense in relation to the child's condition but in terms of breach of parental duties. Are these parental duties described over-ambitiously, given the economic and social realities of most developing countries? Might child protection laws, *expressly* defining child abuse, including sexual abuse, and providing resources for family support, rehabilitation and child refuge centres, be better mechanisms for prevention and detection?

In a few jurisdictions, notably Scandinavia, corporal punishment, whether inflicted at home or at school, is considered child abuse. The Swedish Parliament passed a law in January 1979 which prohibits parents using physical punishment in correcting their children. Norway passed similar legislation in 1980; there corporal punishment in schools had been outlawed as early as 1891. More Western countries are now accepting that corporal punishment should not be sanctioned, but to lay down a law everywhere that a parent cannot lay a finger on a child is probably a counsel of perfection without hope of implementation. It should be remembered that in Sweden and Norway the education of parents and teachers on the wisdom and philosophy of non-violent child correction took many years; it is encouraging that child-abuse cases are extremely rare in those countries, supporting the way to similar legislative moves elsewhere.

In Britain, a few (30 out of 125) local education authorities have instructed schools in their areas to ban corporal punishment, but they cannot enforce the ban in voluntary-aided schools (mostly church), where it continues. Caning is banned in most community homes (for children in care); a few allow smacking rather than caning, or vice versa. Judicial caning as a sentence from the Juvenile Courts has been banned since an Isle of Man case was adjudicated by the European Court. Almost every European country has banned corporal punishment in schools by legislation; Britain is an exception.

In developing countries, particularly those who have inherited British juridical systems, corporal punishment is not considered as a form of child abuse, and judicial caning persists. As we have seen, some civil and family codes authorize parents to inflict "moderate" punishment, but what is viewed as "moderate" is not stated.

The social sanctioning of corporal punishment, particularly in Britain and much of the English-speaking world and its ex-colonies, clearly has links with the battering of children at home. Few authorities writing on child abuse do not acknowledge this connection[7]. Certainly it is significant that in cultures where physical punishment of children is not sanctioned (these are admittedly few in number) child abuse is not thought to take place on anything like the scale that it does in Britain. A definition of child abuse which accommodates corporal punishment, as exists in Scandinavian countries, although not capable immediately of changing child-rearing practices, could provide a useful means of educating parents and society about the dangers of child violence in the home. Much abuse of children is the result of corporal punishment which has gone wrong — either the result of deliberate action causing more harm than was intended or the product of loss of self-control. Either way, the legal definition of this type of abusive behaviour should concern itself with the behaviour itself, and not its consequences or its motivation. The British House of Commons Select Committee on Child Abuse, in 1977, refused to include corporal punishment in its discussions; in like vein the United States Supreme Court in 1977 upheld the constitutionality of corporal punishment in schools. In effect, the Court held that a severe beating by a teacher was not "cruel" within the terms of the Constitution. However, a doctor failing to report the bruises under mandatory reporting arrangements would risk an action for negligence. This is not the only paradox in definitions of abuse, for a court might well uphold the removal of a child from his parents for the very same "abuse" which schools have a licence to carry out.

The definition of child abuse in national legislation can thus be seen to have political, social, and moral overtones, and to reflect the concerns of professional interest groups and the community at large. While every country must define child abuse and neglect as appropriate to its culture and legislative systems, it must seem that child protection laws should cover at least the following:

    a)   Physical injury, if (i) it is known, admitted, or reasonably suspected that the injury was inflicted by any person having care of the child; (ii) any such person knowingly failed to prevent the injury or acted without due regard to the child's safety; (iii) the nature of the injury is inconsistent with the account of how it occurred.

b) Physical neglect, such as the persistent or severe exposure of the child to danger (e.g., cold or starvation) which results in serious impairment of the child's health and development, or failure to thrive which is medically diagnosed as non-organic.

d) Emotional abuse, that is the persistent rejection, hostility, coldness of a parent or guardian towards a child which has severe effects on the child's behaviour and development. In some cases, over-protectiveness on the part of the carer may also have an adverse effect.

e) Sexual abuse, being the involvement of a child with a parent or carer in any form of sexual activity to which the child cannot give consent by law or because of ignorance, dependence, development immaturity or fear.

f) Extra-familial abuse, including exploitation of the child in the labour market, in detrimental ritutal practices, in trafficking, in begging, prostitution, etc.

Clearly "harm" goes beyond deliberate maltreatment by parents, but where can the line be drawn? In the poorest countries, children are subjected continually to malnutrition and exploitation, and even to torture and imprisonment. The ignorance, poverty and homelessness of parents creates a situation in which the child is inevitably neglected; however, the neglect is no fault of the family but, rather, the result of extreme underdevelopment and the environment.

To conclude, there can be no satisfactory clear definition of child abuse to fit all countries and all purposes. We can only indicate the general contours of the concept of child abuse. When legislative approaches to child abuse are discussed below, attention will be focused on what the procedures are in developed countries and in relation mainly to intra-familial abuse.

ILO Conventions[8] and national laws should cover extra-familial abuse such as child labour, child prostitution, trafficking, child marriages, and vagrancy. Children on plantations should also enjoy the protection of the general laws affecting all young persons. These laws are as yet poorly implemented, owing to weak law-enforcement machinery and lack of political will. They are concerned mostly with the punishment of the offenders, not with the welfare of the exploited child. (Often financial penalties are unrealistically low and rarely recovered, and corruption is rife). Laws need formulation which promote child welfare in general whether the abuse comes from within the family or from outside in the wider society; definitions of abuse should make the coverage clear.

IDENTIFICATION AND REPORTING OF CHILD ABUSE

Recognizing child abuse is a function of its definition, of course, in that the broader the definition adopted by the law the easier it is recognized. The negative side of the broad legally effective definition is that the State may intervene excessively, and oppressively.

Child abuse must be identifiable by features which those with a trained competence — such as the police, social workers, doctors, health visitors, teachers — and the public at large — neighbours, other children, and people active in the locality such as milkmen (UK) and tradesmen—can recognize.

Of course, it is the professionals who must be considered in the forefront of the identification team, but the general public must also be educated and informed about the existence and meaning of child abuse, and to whom they can report it confidentially. In the United States[9], since the 1970s, all the states have had a system of mandatory reporting, and this is a rapidly evolving field of law. Most of these reporting statutes have been amended in significant respects once or several times during the 1970s and will continue to evolve to reflect developments in research, casework practice and states' experience in administering child protection systems. Whether state welfare systems have the resources to respond to the volume of reported cases is another question. "The enactment of a reporting statute is foolish business unless reported children are in fact protected from further injury and offered a chance of a brighter life either within the family or with other people, should remaining at home prove impossible" commented one legal scholar[10] on this issue.

The problem initially when mandatory reporting for doctors was first discussed was the confidentiality that exists with the patient: physicians' resistance to statutory reporting was initially high since many considered that disclosure to the authorities of their suspicions of abuse or neglect would constitute an ethical or legal breach of the professional relationship. However, the reporting statutes either expressly or implicitly abrogate the confidential nature of the disclosure and whatever privileged status it may have under the legal rules of evidence. Reporting is designed to promote the welfare of the patient, who is, of course, the child. A physician who does not report a suspected case in any case might find himself the defendant in civil or criminal proceedings for negligence, and for breach of his duty of care to the child patient. The doctor must clearly favour protection of a child over protection of the confidentiality of its suspected or potential assailant.

In Holland, doctors were similarly reluctant to report cases of child abuse; the difficulties were avoided by a novel approach. The doctor may report his suspicions about child abuse to his district *Vertranensate* (confidential doctor), who is part of a multi-disciplinary team which includes a social worker and a coordinator. Because the family doctor is in first contact with another professional colleague he feels less responsible for breaking the confidentiality of the relationship with the suspected abuser.

In Britain, there is no system of mandatory reporting but all local authorities maintain at-risk registers. The prime purpose of the register is to safeguard children from abuse by providing a record of those who are believed to have been victims of abuse or about whom serious concern is already felt. The register is made up of two parts: active and inactive. The second list contains the names of children who have been deregistered and also names of adults known to have been involved with child abuse. Registration does not constitute legal proof that child abuse has taken place, but records concern and anxiety.

In recent months, in the wake of an unusually high number of child abuse cases which have led to deaths, there have been a number of attempts to widen the types of personnel who should be acquainted with child abuse. For example, the Inner London Education Authority has issued directives to all its schools asking that all teachers should be on the look-out for signs of maltreatment. Fairly detailed procedures have been adopted, involving in the protection system the ordinary class teacher along with the head-teacher, the social services, the police, and the education welfare officer system. The class teacher is advised to take steps, even on her own, to contact the education welfare officer, if it is felt that the head-teacher is not taking any action. In some areas of the country, the milkmen (who deliver bottled milk daily in nearly every home) have been recruited to assist in detecting and reporting child abuse, since they see families every morning regularly and may notice changes in the appearance of children on the doorsteps. In Manchester, the City Council has set up a special unit in the police force. Hospitals are beginning to develop specialist teams.

Self-reporting also has a role to play in child abuse, but to be feasible it requires the consequence of reporting to be non-penal and therapeutic, aimed at helping the self-reporting abusing guardian to face his problems and accept assistance. The problem in legislation on reporting is whether it should be mandatory or voluntary; and whether all persons should be bound to report suspected child abuse (with due protection of their confidentiality) or only selected professionals. Another possibility is to bind none and encourage everyone. Some Canadian jurisdictions have mandatory reporting, and others contain uncertain obligations. The Ontario Child Welfare Act is anomalous: it provides that "every person having information of the abandonment, desertion, physical ill-treatment or need of protection of a child shall report the information to a children's aid society or Crown Attorney. Notwithstanding that the information is confidential or privileged, no action shall be instituted against the informant unless the giving of the information is done maliciously or without reasonable and probable cause". This statute gives no sanction for failure to report. Section 41 of the Quebec *Youth Protection Act* (1981) binds any adult to bring the necessary assistance to a child who wishes to alert the authorities of his or any other child's danger, and provides such adults with immunity from prosecution, if the reporting was done in good faith.

It is obviously essential that any report, from whatever source, about child abuse should be immediately investigated by the social services or the police. The murder of seven-year-old Maria Colwell, the subject of a public enquiry in Britain in 1974[11], might never have happened if social workers had taken seriously the complaints of neighbours who were concerned about the little girl's terrible appearance some weeks before she died at the hands of her stepfather. There have been cases where a social worker has disbelieved a colleague's independent expression of concern, and a tragedy has resulted. Yet self-reporting and reporting of child abuse by ordinary citizens may not occur if those giving information fear that the immediate consequence for the abuser will be criminal prosecution and imprisonment. If the consequence of investigation that confirmed that suspicion were known to be treatment, support, and assistance to the family and the child, more children might be protected and greater abuse prevented.

When reporting is obligatory by law, the existence of penal sanctions for breach of this statutory duty provides a convenient excuse for those who do stand in some relationship of trust and confidentiality with the suspected abuser. "I should be prosecuted if I did not report" the reporter (social worker or neighbour) can explain should the need arise.

115

Mandatory reporting should be introduced in all countries where child abuse is a problem. The list of professional people bound by the legal duty might include teachers, doctors, health visitors, nurses, and extension and community workers. All doctors should be educated on the medical aspects of child abuse, for laws would require a medical diagnosis as well as a social assessment.

Doctors who treat child prostitutes in Bombay for venereal disease, rape, and other abuses rarely report these appalling cases, owing to reluctance to become involved with the police and courts. A system of compulsory reporting, with penal sanctions, would help to ensure that these girl prostitutes, many of them kidnapped in Nepal and objects of multiple re-sales, were rescued, treated and rehabilitated. Mandatory reporting on these matters would assist in the implementation of national legislation (in line with ILO Conventions) on the *Prohibition of Immoral Traffic of Women and Girls,* a penal law on the statute books of many countries, but poorly enforced. Such a legislative move might also pave the way for better liaison between doctors and police so that the struggle to abolish child prostitution would have some chance of success. The acceptance or offering of bribes to stop the reporting could be prohibited with maximum punishment. The Indian Health Association is working to achieve legislation. The same approach could be used in respect of other abusive practices such as female circumcision and the cruel treatment, torture and murder of child brides over the dowry. In India, Bangladesh and Sri Lanka, laws in theory impose heavy penalties for rape, dowry threats and cruelty[12] but doctors seem reluctant to report and testify. Mandatory reporting, on the US lines, could be introduced in other areas of extra-familial abuse such as child labour in factories and unlicensed workshops; in sex tourism; and in familial exploitation of children in beggary and domestic service.

Children, being vulnerable, inarticulate, isolated and powerless would enjoy greater protection if such laws were passed, although mandatory reporting alone is not enough. Its effectiveness depends upon immediate appropriate action such as removal of the child, a case conference, judicial review, or further investigations. Adequate resources for effective action must be allocated. Public enquiries in Britain which have followed the deaths of children already on at-risk registers or in care have revealed too often a lack of follow-up after reporting, and weak coordination between the various organizations. Professional disciplining of social workers after a tragedy hardly helps the battered child, but a well-publicized system of legislated criminal sanctions on reporting might. Such legislation would indicate more clearly society's decision that child abuse is not private or domestic misconduct but a grave matter calling for public scrutiny and the intervention of the state.

Criminal sanctions on reporting would educate, direct and reinforce good intentions. The publicizing of any prosecutions in the media and professional journals would increase awareness among professionals and the public. Many professionals are reluctant to report suspected child abuse cases because of their unwillingness to become involved with lawyers and the courts. If not to report meant possible criminal prosecution, then more cases would come to light in time to protect the child. A legal obligation to report would also reduce the abuser's resentment and the reporter's embarrassment — an important consideration where the relationship between these two should continue after the event (for example, a social worker or doctor). In the U.S.A. it has become compulsory for an increasing number of health-care professionals to report[13]. Each country must decide how wide or how restricted the list of persons should be. Finally, the definition of "abuse" for the purposes of the reporting law may be somewhat broader than that used for the purposes of administrative or judicial intervention. The agency to receive reports will be determined by the reporting law, but its decision is not a matter of legal significance. In Britain the NSPCC is normally the agency to respond to alarms; teachers report to the education welfare authorities. There may be an argument for limiting compulsory reporting to child welfare agencies, rather than to the police, for the latter may be unwilling to take action if they do not think the evidence justifies a prosecution, or they may make decisions on prosecution strictly by criminal evidence laws. Punishment for non-reporting would need to be decided within the scope of the general law and social policy in each jurisdiction.

MANAGEMENT OF CHILD ABUSE

There have been over 25 formal inquiries into child abuse cases in Britain since the Graham Bagnall case in 1972[14]. The public inquiry into the death of Jasmine Bedford at the hands of her stepfather has just been completed this year[15]. Several well-publicized criminal trials of parents and stepparents have taken place. As each new tragedy is reported in the media, the critical reaction is to blame the social worker in charge of the case. A lack of co-ordination between police, health visitors, the NSPCC, and the schools is frequently shown up. After such publicity there is usually a dramatic reaction in the handling of "non-accidental injury": local authorities concerned to avoid further "mistakes" move, understandably, towards a policy of "removing" more children who are "at risk", which may not always be in the "best interests of the child". To take away a child to an institution or a foster-home may not necessarily be in the "best interests": what may be needed is better support for the family so that it can stay together. The "at-risk register" is not a panacea, but it is a useful working-tool. It is also a preventive measure. Below some other responses are described.

The case-conference

Any professional person who is concerned about a child's safety and convenes a case-conference should be able to communicate directly with the heads of social service agencies or with other suitable bodies in the local area. All those involved with the child should be able to attend the conference, including the parents and the child, depending on the child's age and the circumstances. There has often been discussion within social-work circles about the wisdom of involving the police at this stage; arguments against are based on concern that once the police are involved then, in serious cases, a criminal prosecution is inevitable and therefore work to support and contain the family is immediately frustrated. A successful experiment has been conducted in Northampton, Britain, whereby the chief constable of police is called in at an early stage to cooperate with the medical and legal teams. The "principle of opportunity" exists in many jurisdictions whereby the police are free to decide whether or not to invoke the criminal law; if they have early discussions with social services, they may agree to postpone prosecution in the child's interests. At the same time, the involvement of the police at the outset with their forensic expertise is useful in collecting evidence for any future civil "care" proceedings, since their evidence will not be easily refuted by the cross-examination of astute lawyers acting for the parent.

The composition, terms of reference, and powers of case-conferences could be written into child-protection legislation, as well as the period of time within which there must be reviews of the situation of the child and the family, whether the child is at home or with foster-parents or in institutional care. In Sweden the Law of 1980 states that care provisions must be renewed every six months. Coordination between all agencies and professionals through the case-conferences could be written into child protection laws.

JUDICIAL RESPONSES TO CHILD ABUSE

(i) *Penal responses*

Every physical abuse of a child constitutes an offence against the person and can be prosecuted under the general criminal law. Laws lay down the specific penalties for certain acts against children; others leave the question of punishment to the courts but may state maximum and minimum penalties. The varieties of child abuse afford various choices. The gravest offences — such as murder — attract the highest penalty. Other offences may be viewed in different lights according to whether the act is one of a series or an isolated incident, the abuser is willing to obtain treatment, there are social circumstances which have contributed to the criminal behaviour and which may be improved by social assistance, or the abuser may be safely given a suspended sentence and kept under supervision, thus keeping the family intact.

Psychologists have reported on the severe trauma experienced by abused children giving evidence against parents or other family members in criminal trials. Still to be resolved is how to deal with the uncorroborated evidence of the very young witness. In Britain and elsewhere the uncorroborated evidence of a child under the age of seven is not admissible. An approach explored in some 11 American state legal systems is to make a tape- or video-recording of the child's evidence, to avoid the child having to attend the adult criminal court. The alleged abuser faced with such recorded evidence may confess to the crime, avoiding the need of a long-drawn-out contested case. Lawyers in some jurisdictions will find this experiment repugnant because it contravenes the fundamental rules of natural justice, coercing the accused into admission, and not allowing a cross-examination of the child. In an Australian state the abuser may be tried and sentenced in the juvenile court, where the environment and procedures are less disturbing for the child witness, and where the court can make some alternative dispositions, with the child and family's welfare as the paramount consideration.

In many jurisdictions the exercise of prosecutorial discretion is becoming a feature of the administration of the criminal law. If so, then (with good liaison with the police) it may be agreed that, in the child's interests, a criminal

118

prosecution should not be brought but the matter considered in civil proceedings in the juvenile or family court.

Certain jurisdictions contain special penal provisions relating to distinct offences — sex crimes, for example. The penalties may be greater, depending on the victim's age. Child prostitution may be regarded as "statutory" rape. In several Latin-American countries trafficking and prostitution of young girls is an increasing social problem but as yet not governed by any special penal provisions. Specific penal laws might help to protect these abused street-children and protect others. By contrast, in Bangladesh the Cruelty to Women (Deterrent Punishment) Ordinance, of 1983, covers such acts as kidnapping and abduction of women for unlawful or immoral purposes. The punishment is transportation for life (an inheritance surely of the old British colonial penal law) or a "rigorous" term of imprisonment for up to 14 years, and a fine. Trafficking causing death for dowry reasons, and rape or attempted rape of minors, carry distinct penal sanctions, but the law is barely enforced and few prosecutions have been brought before the courts. In India the same is true, where the Suppression of Immoral Traffic Act for Women and Girls (1956), and the Prevention of Devadasi Act, 1981, on temple prostitution have failed to have much effect on the sexual corruption of minors[16].

In developing countries many factors impede the enforcement of laws aimed at protecting children: lack of resources, police reluctance to intervene, and the possibility of corruption where the punishment is merely a fine. Delays in bringing cases to trial result in the disappearance of important prosecution witnesses. A much publicized case of the prostitution of a 12-year-old Nepalese girl illustrates this point. The suspected brothel owners were arrested and bailed but two years later they still have not been tried. The child may prove a weak witness in view of the delay. Often the accused break bail and cannot be traced. Arguably, for certain serious offences of child abuse, no bail should be given, and in all cases where charges are laid the trial should take place as soon as possible. A child's memory is short; the trauma of giving evidence is in itself a damaging experience, and the criminal proceedings should be completed as quickly as possible.

The powers of sentencing in the criminal courts in many countries rarely include sending the offender for treatment. It may be that for certain types of child abuse — sexual exploitation and excessive regimes — there should be room for such a course. In all but the most serious cases, the criminal law appears a blunt tool for treating child abuse within the family. In theory, adults who assault their own children should be treated like any other assailant, but the strict approach does not achieve its purpose. First, it may be impossible to isolate abuse from the total family situation; second, the child may be better off with the family under supervision than anywhere else; third, criminal prosecution divides families and buries the child in guilt that can create far more permanent damage than the original incident or incidents. Fourth, if there is a danger of prosecution, a parent or carer may fear the consequences of seeking treatment for an injured child. Fifth, time spent in penal custody will not prepare the abuser to meet the demands of family life after release. And finally, in case of acquittal the accused carer may regard it as legitimizing his behaviour, and this may make supervision of the family and further social work difficult to maintain. Here again, it is impossible to make any statement which will have global application: different cultures will have their own views about the offence, punishment and family circumstances, and much will depend upon the resources available to put in process alternative sentencing and arrangements for therapies and supervision.

(ii) *Civil proceedings for child protection*

Protection or care proceedings need not be contentious, but they often are. The "adversarial" approach is used in order to protect the parent and family as much as the child. Care proceedings are often "three-handers", with the local authority or child welfare organization embattled with the parents and the child over custody, care and control. It may develop into a contest between the lawyers, and the true "best interests" of the child are buried under court procedures and legal argument. The establishment of family courts, or specially trained juvenile court justices to handle care cases, is becoming a feature of an increasing number of jurisdictions, and may go some way to defuse the "adversary" atmosphere.

(a) Place-of-Safety Order

In most developed countries, when a child is shown to be in need of care and protection there are certain actions than can be taken. If a child has been seriously injured or a social worker, doctor, police officer, or other person suspects that the child is in immediate danger, there are procedures for emergency action. In Britain a Place-of-Safety Order (PSO) (s.28 Children and Young Persons Act) can be sought immediately, either through the Juvenile Court or, outside court hours, at the residence of any magistrate, who must be satisfied that the reporter has reasonable cause to suspect that a serious injury has occurred or might occur if a Place-of-Safety Order were not made. An Order is often taken out after a child is admitted to hospital with a suspected non-accidental injury. The grounds for obtaining an order to remove the child or detain him or her in hospital are not as strict as those for a full-care order. "Reasonable suspicion" is sufficient. The authorities need time to investigate the case more fully. In theory, the order may be granted for up to 28 days, but in practice magistrates grant it for the shortest possible time so that the parties can come to court, where the local authority must argue its case under the Children and Young Persons Act.

The Place-of-Safety Order having been obtained, the authorities must decide, after further inquiries, whether to apply to the court for a full care order, an interim care order or a supervision order, or to allow the case to be monitored outside the remit of the court. Much will depend upn the weight of evidence the authorities can muster.

(b) Proposals for a 'child production order'

In Britain, a glaring loophole in child protection law was recently revealed at the trial of a stepfather who starved a three-year-old girl to death. Social workers and health visitors had attempted to see the child reported to be at risk, but were deceived by lies and excuses: the child was "asleep", "ill", "out", or "staying with grandparents" or "visiting friends". Because there is no intermediate power between a mere enquiry and a Place-of-Safety Order, nothing could be done. A simple legal change proposed is the introduction of a "child production order", obtainable from a magistrate confidentially (to protect informants) by social workers, police or other professionals upon sworn evidence. Such an order would require a named person (usually a parent) to produce a named child for inspection. Such an innovation would not constitute an infringement of civil liberties, since no crime is alleged or punishment imposed.

Alternatively, all children under five years (that is, below compulsory school age and thus more vulnerable) could be monitored regularly at maternal and child health clinics. Failure to keep appointments could trigger off home visits, and the "child production order" if the professional failed to see the child.

(c) Care proceedings

Where care cases come before the courts, the child welfare agencies will usually have prepared reports on the abuse, and on all the relevant family circumstances. In English law, under the Children and Young Persons Act, two matters must be proved: first, that the child has been a victim of abuse, and, second, that if the court does not make an order the child will be without proper care and control. Both these matters must be adjudicated on the civil test of proof — on the balance of probabilities, not, as in criminal proceedings, beyond all reasonable doubt, whereas in the criminal trials of alleged abusers the criminal standard of proof applies. Thus an abuser might be acquitted in the criminal court under the penal law, yet in the civil court the case is proved. The principal difference is that in the criminal court the abuser is on trial, whereas in the civil proceedings what is at issue is the paramount welfare of the child. After finding the case proved, the court may, after reading the welfare reports, find that already recent social work intervention has resulted in a change of circumstances. The parents are prepared to seek help, or have been shocked by the initiation of care proceedings into changing their behaviour, or the abuser has left the family home or is in prison for the offence and will not be returning in the foreseeable future. The court may decide that rather than a care order a supervision order is appropriate; or it may decide to make no order at all, having satisfied itself that the local authority's plans for the child, on a voluntary basis, are a guarantee against future harm.

(d) Guardian *ad Litem*

In Britain, in contested care matters, the parties are the local authority and the child, and until this year parents were not parties to the proceedings, although at the discretion of the court they could make a statement and cross-examine witnesses who made allegations against them. Since implementation of certain provisions of the Child Care Act, 1980, parents now can be quasi-parties to care proceedings. But where the parents seek to discharge a care order and in all cases of suspected non-accidental-injury, or where there is conflict between the child and parent in contested care proceedings, the child must be separately represented by a "guardian *ad litem*".* This is not a servant of the court but an independent lawyer or social worker who can investigate the circumstances of the case and act wholly in the child's interests.

Most Family Courts in New York automatically appoint guardians *ad litem* to represent the child in all neglect proceedings if such an arrangement is

---

* Guardian appointed for a lawsuit.

applicable. A child's advocate is chosen from a special panel, whose members are sufficiently knowledgeable about children and have undergone some special training.

In some jurisdictions the child may not be an active party in any proceedings to take away parental rights: the contest is between the parents and the state. This seems to be the position in many developing countries: in Cuba, Bolivia, the Philippines, and Brazil, where family and civil codes lay down the conditions of *patria potestas.* The child cannot be a party. But should the child be able to establish a right to be represented, as in delinquency cases, a guardian *ad litem* could protect him from excesses of state and parents. The law tends to presume that a child's parents are best suited to represent him against the intervention of the authorities. Yet the child needs protection from unjustified state interference in his upbringing as he does from abuse by parents. Although clearly parents should not represent their children when their fitness as carers is under scrutiny, the plans of the state or local authority for the child may be equally detrimental to its proper development, by being kept in an institution, fostering, changes in type and place of care or lack of continuity. It is not enough for the child to be represented by a lawyer, for the latter may be taking instructions from the parent, where the abused child is too young to give instructions personally.

British laws finally caught up with American and some Canadian law in 1985. It could be argued that in all countries where cases of child abuse occur a guardian *ad litem* should be appointed. If lawyers for the child are instructed by the parent in abuse cases, it is tantamount to the prosecution, in a criminal matter, taking instructions from the defendant.

(e) Adversarial or inquisitorial

Care proceedings usually take place in juvenile or family courts, but they may be heard in ordinary civil courts, or in criminal courts along with the prosecution of the offender. Care proceedings might be better managed if they were non-adversary, non-party proceedings. They should never be seen as a contest between the state, the parents, and the child or their respective lawyers. They should be an objective enquiry into all matters pertaining to the child, with the object of reaching a decision which is in its "best interests" or, as Goldstein, Freud and Solnit suggest, "the least detrimental" to the child[17]. The ordinary rules on the admissibility of evidence should be relaxed so that hearsay evidence is admissible. (In the Maria Colwell case the public enquiry following her death heard that she had cried bitterly on learning she was to be removed from her foster parents, but the lawyer representing her took instructions from her mother, who wanted her at home, and this evidence was never presented at the care proceedings. It was the child's solicitor who was able to use the hearsay prohibition rule to protect the mother and her cohabitee, who later killed the child).

It may be that all abuse and neglect proceedings should be held in two stages: adjudication and dispositional, as in New York State and Scotland. In Scotland, children's panels consider in an informal setting what is in the child's best interests, after the adversary process has dealt with the issue of whether the abuse occurred and whether a court order should be made. The panel is composed of lay people with experience, knowledge and understanding of children. The key is the "reporter", who may be a lawyer or a social worker or both. The panel can review all the earlier decisions and question the social worker about plans for the future. It is not a court and does not merely rubber-stamp social services' decisions, like some juvenile and family courts. Some juvenile courts in Inner London have experimented with "moving the furniture" in the courtroom, so that all the decisions relating to the child's future can be discussed in a relaxed way "around a table" rather than in the cold and formal setting of a tribunal. The judge or justices, if the procedure is inquisitorial, can feel free to ask questions of the social services as to what their plans are for the future — whether they are planning rehabilitation with the family, long-term fostering or adoption, and what access there will be if the child is removed from home. They can call for a review after a fixed period. By this process the delicate relationship between social worker and the family is more likely to be preserved, an important consideration where the worker must continue to support the family even where, on the social worker's evidence, a decision to withdraw parental rights is made.

In the United States, Canada, Great Britain and other developed countries, the suitability of the traditional adversarial system of trial procedure to resolve child protection applications has been doubted, not least because of the excessive delays to which it is subject and the partisan atmosphere of trial. Law reform commissions might consider exploring the feasibility of alternative procedures on the models of those countries that have already established other systems. A judicial decision concerning a family, reached in amicable consensus in an informal family court, promises a better outcome than one reached amid bitter conflict. Protection proceedings need not be contentious; ways can be found to safeguard the parents' rights while putting the child's interest foremost.

The link between law and social services

Each time a terrible tragedy of child abuse and neglect hits the headlines, it is often the social workers who are pilloried — criticized for not having foreseen the degree of risk in their concern to keep their client's family intact, or rebuked for actions that have fragmented a family and forced a removal of the child. In Britain, public enquiries reveal some of the problems: poor coordination between supervisors and juniors in the social services; overlapping and duplication of responsibilities; too many agencies involved; overburdening case-loads and underqualified personnel; and bad pay and conditions. As moral outrage and panic grows with each new reported case of child ill-treatment, social workers understandably may rush to "defensive" action and remove children to what may not necessarily be better in the long run for the child. When courts make supervision orders, instead of a requested care order, there is public panic if the decision turns out to be ill-advised. Yet social workers cannot be on duty 24 hours a day within the privacy of a child's home. Some commentators feel that all social workers will always try to resist a removal order, since such action implies their failure to succeed with family case-work, and an order once made destroys any relationship built up with clients, with whom they must continue to work whatever the decision. Others argue that social workers wish to "control" and "interfere" in family life, that they are interfering, and make subjective judgements. Often what is crucial to the welfare of families is the total environment, over which the social worker can have no influence, such as housing, education, amenities, employment and financial support. In court the social worker is pulled in opposite directions: her duty to the parent conflicts with that to the child and the court. Sometime her evidence is discredited by the court, demolished in cross-examination by astute lawyers.

The relationship between lawyers and social workers, like that between lawyers and doctors, is understandably fraught with problems in communication and allegiances. It is imperative that each profession be trained in the other's basic principles. In addition, social workers need to be trained to explain the functions of the judiciary to their clients, while keeping open access to them. Lawyers and judges need to understand better the constraints that social workers invariably encounter in their work. Joint seminars for members of the different professions could be a useful means of ironing out the difficulty in communication, and ensure that social reports and verbal evidence are provided in a manner fit for the courts.

Civil and criminal liability of social workers

Over the past 10 years the potential civil and criminal liability of social workers has become an unavoidable element in child welfare work in the United States, and this could occur also in Britain and elsewhere. In the USA there have been dozens of civil lawsuits and criminal proceedings against child welfare workers and their agencies. In Britain, in September of this year, a senior inspector of the National Society for the Prevention of Cruelty to Children (NSPCC), the largest and most important voluntary organization helping children, entered a false report in case records about seeing a three-year-old girl alive and well. In fact, the child was already dead, having been starved over a period of several months. The inspector, apparently suffering from domestic stress at the time, was immediately dismissed. In the USA he would have faced criminal prosecution.

Yet, setting aside such incidents of deliberate malpractice, every year children suffer further maltreatment or death *after* their plight becomes known to a protective agency. Studies in Britain and a number of states in the USA show that about a quarter of all child deaths attributed to abuse and neglect involve children already reported to, or under the care of, a protective agency. Tens of thousands of other children receive serious injuries short of death while under child protective supervision. Since proceedings are normally confidential, relatively few of these cases are reported in the media. But those that do attract publicity tend to have an impact on social workers and social work practice beyond what their number would suggest. At the same time there is no publicity for social-work practice and decision-making that has turned out ultimately to benefit the child.

As a result there is a tendency to blame individual case-workers for deaths. In the USA, in addition to professional disciplining, groups of social workers have been criminally prosecuted for official malfeasance and negligent homicide or called before investigating grand juries.

If social workers have been careless or negligent it is right that they should bear the blame. But in many cases no one could have prevented a child's death, since even the most experienced social worker cannot predict the future behaviour of individual parents. First, a social worker's decisions are based on information which may be incomplete, inaccurate or misleading. It is almost impossible for even the most skilled investigator to find out what really happened in a case of child abuse occurring in the privacy of the home, unless the child is old enough or brave enough to speak out or another family member comes forward. Second, staff shortages and heavy case-loads limit the level of supervision. Third, home conditions can deteriorate very suddenly and without warning. Emergency action to remove a child is justified when a serious injury has already happened, but, unless the parent is suffering from a severe and demonstrable mental illness, even the best clinician would be unable to make a reliable judgement about the parent's propensity to be abusive or neglectful.

Regrettably, however laws are framed and administrative arrangements shaped, social workers can never "guarantee" the safety of all children reported to them. They can only do their best. Too much power to social workers to intervene can, as we have warned earlier, be equally damaging to a child's proper development. Unbridled criticism of social workers, the threat of prosecution, and dismissal can lead to "defensive" social work. Social workers feel they will be blamed if there was any reason, however minute, for suspecting that a child was in danger. Accordingly they may try to get "care orders" for all suspected abused children, to protect themselves from professional censure or criminal prosecution. In the three years following Maria Colwell's death in Britain, the number of place-of-safety orders increased three and a half times. Such a state of affairs is not good for the children or the families or the social-work profession. Better laws could remedy this situation.

How laws can assist social work

Most countries have legislation which provides some broad indications of what is considered abusive or neglectful parental behaviour, giving grounds for the state to remove the child. But their vagueness and breadth may delegate too much power to the state through its administrators and case-workers in child protection agencies. They may give social workers too broad an authority to intervene, while poor legal drafting inhibits their ability to make their case before a court. Existing laws could be reviewed to see whether redrafting could provide better protection for the social worker by stating more precisely the situations in which immediate removal is essential, for example, where a parent has acted in a way that had caused serious injury, was capable of causing serious injury or, if continued over time, would cause serious injury. Laws could be redrafted to make clear that the only justified basis for removal is the parent's *past* behaviour, with two exceptions: where a parent suffers from a severe and proven mental illness, and where a parent through "self-reporting" has expressed fear of hurting or killing a child. Laws could exempt social workers from legal liability except where criminal negligence could be proved. Legal and administrative changes will not remove from social workers the burden of having to make borderline decisions. In addition to removals, they are confronted with the decisions of when to return a child to parents after a period in care, or whether to continue supervision or close the case entirely. In the case of Maria Colwell the social worker decided to return the child to the mother because the mother wanted the child back; no one listened to the child's views or checked on Maria's stepfather. Anyone who did so would have recognized Maria's terror at the prospect of return and discovered that the stepfather had a criminal record for violence. Fortunately, lessons were learnt from that tragedy. Now children like Maria have independent legal guardians, and the names of child-abusers may be kept on an at-risk register.

Social workers are criticized sharply when children are killed when supposedly under their supervision or care, or labelled as authoritarian and interventionist when they apply to the courts for judicial orders or otherwise interfere in the family. This criticism is unfair and leads to less good social work. Social work professionals should be partners with lawyers in formulating child protective legislation which would improve the efficiency of both the legal and the caring professions. The suggested Child Production Order is only one example of a possible legal reform.

Public inquiries

In Britain, numerous public inquiries have followed child-abuse deaths. However, the social work professions question the wisdom of scrutinizing these tragedies in public. The Jasmine Bedford inquiry held this year cost the taxpayer between £120,000 and £1 million; according to an NSPCC spokesman, this was "more than will be spent on training in child abuse through the rest of the country this year". Such sums could be better spent on family support schemes and improving the environment. Apart from the length and cost, other obligations are their general effect on the social workers involved and the profession in general, and the lack of any satisfactory outcome of such inquiries. The series of inquiries tread similar ground, with little effect on main policy issues. Moreover, the public probing of social workers by lawyers more accustomed to criminal court trials casts the social workers in the role of defendants and has affected relationships both between the professionals and between them and their clients.

The Maria Colwell enquiry did produce important changes in child care law, and as a result of the Aukland inquiry in 1975 social service departments must now be informed of the release of any persons convicted of offences against children in their area. Also the law on care proceedings has been tightened. The child must be provided with a guardian *ad litem*. These have been important improvements. Yet there is a strong case for insisting that inquiries be held in private: social workers giving evidence would be protected from the distorted reporting of the media, which often pillory them unmercifully. Social workers invariably have to take risks with the future welfare of children and should rightly be accountable to the public, but public enquiries may prove to have more damaging effects, offsetting their potential usefulness in identifying the real issues. Among these are the quality of social work practice; development of skills and training; coordination between different professionals and agencies; the loopholes in present laws which need filling. The sad result of this type of publicity is that social workers, fearful in the wake of such tragedies, tend to recommend more removals then before, and judges too, mindful of events, are similarly influenced. The social worker's responsibility is immense, as is that of the lawyer, the guardian *ad litem*, and the court. All that responsible persons can hope to achieve is "the least detrimental available alternative for safeguarding the child's development". However, social workers cannot be expected to be on 24-hours surveillance of families; nor, if it were possible, would such continual vigilance do other than seriously damage the family's self-esteem and capacity to cope.

126

CONCLUSION AND RECOMMENDATIONS

International and national concern over the alarming increase in abused and neglected children has led many countries to pass new laws. In some jurisdictions special laws on child abuse have been enacted as part of the criminal law; in others, the general criminal law pertains, and the legal protection of abused children is covered by child protection acts and the civil courts. Basically, the laws are concerned with procedures.

Child abuse and neglect, however, do not occur only within families, but extrafamilial forms have not been dealt with in this paper, for the subject would then be too broad to cover. Child prostitution, trafficking, forced marriages, exploitative illegal labour, and degrading treatment call for more effective ways of enforcing national laws. ILO Conventions address many of these activities and should be reflected in domestic legislation. Education of the community on both the existence of types of abuse and the prohibiting laws might encourage better reporting and consequent arrests of offenders and rescue of the children concerned. The following recommendations might be adapted to individual jurisdictions as appropriate:

General recommendations

1. The establishment by legislation of either a minister for children or a children's ombudsman (on the Swedish and Norwegian model), with a campaigning, educational, law-reform advisory and policy role.
2. The setting up of family courts to exercise juvenile and family jurisdiction.
3. The establishment of a children's legal centre (on the lines of the Ontario-based "Justice for Children") which could promote nationally the rights of children and increase awareness of them; be a resource centre for individuals, including lawyers; provide legal advice and arrange education and training for lawyers and other professionals concerned.
4. Attachment of a "family impact statement" in all new or proposed legislation and administrative changes[18], to ensure that policies support families and children.
5. Implementation of the spirit of the sections of the Draft Convention on the Rights of the Child related to child abuse.

Recommendations specific to child abuse

The formulation of legislation to cover the following:

1. The establishment of a national child-abuse unit within a government ministry or department (health, social services, or youth) responsible for education and research on child abuse, for advising government, and for training all key workers in its prevention, detection and management.
2. The establishment and maintenance of registers in each locality, providing details of children who are at risk. The establishment of a special register of child-sex offenders (although this might conflict with an offender's right to clearance following sentence or acquittal).

3. The establishment in police stations, hospitals and local authority social service and education departments of special units to deal with child abuse and neglect.
4. Training of personnel in the detection and prevention of child abuse.
5. The inclusion of powers of any court to use alternative disposals for the offender, such as treatment, rehabilitation, counselling, family therapy, or admission to hospital.
6. Allocation of the necessary resources to child welfare agencies, statutory and voluntary.
7. Compulsory education and training of doctors, social workers, teachers, health visitors and police on the handling of child abuse.
8. Legally obliging certain professionals or all members of the public, as appropriate, to report cases of child abuse.
9. "24-hour hotlines" for immediate action on suspected abuse, and special services for handling sexual abuse; and introduction of a "child production" order.
10. Removal of evidentiary obstacles in adjudicating on child-abuse cases and their disposition, e.g., trial of tape-recording of interviews with the child victim, or the admissibility of evidence of the very young child (with suitable precautions).

The above are some broad recommendations. In addition, since child abuse is as much a social problem as one resulting from the abuser's psychopathology, every effort must be made to eliminate the external causal factors. All national policies need to be monitored to ensure that they are not detrimental to the welfare of families. Among the policy options that might be considered most urgent are compulsory education for parenthood; maternity leave for working mothers; family planning services to reach the most disadvantaged, for many abused children are unwanted; day-care centres; crisis refuge centres for children; child allowances to be paid direct to mothers or through mother and children clinics; school counselling services; recreation facilities; guaranteed minimum income for families.

A theory of child abuse that relates it to the environment and poverty does not explain its occurrence in the higher socioeconomic classes, where it is also observed. Nevertheless the sociological interpretation of child abuse must be considered alongside the pathological one. It is, of course, more expensive to tackle the root sources of poverty than to treat the child after the event. However, it is outside the scope of this paper to set down all the ways in which the poverty of children and their families can be tackled: child abuse needs to be tackled on *all* fronts, including the environmental ones, and legislation to improve the environment for children should be consided — hence the importance of a "family impact statement".

Child abuse and neglect is a matter of legal as well as medical and social concern. Only a handful of the legal and juridical issues have been discussed in these pages, and it has been almost impossible to consider these in a way that can have global application. Every country needs to create an effective programme under the law, and the courts must be full partners in such efforts. Constitutional requirements and statutory definitions in most countries so demand it.

Notes

[1] Legislation to protect animals from cruelty was passed in 1823. See Hansard H.C. Vol 337, col 229.

[2] See V. Fontana, *Somewhere a Child is Crying,* London, Macmillan, 1973, and Catherine J. Ross, *The Lessons of the Past: Defining and Controlling Child Abuse in the United States* In: G. Gerbner *et al. Child Abuse.* New York, Oxford University Press. 1980 (pp. 63–81).

[3] H. Kempe. The Battered Baby Syndrome. *Journal of the American Medical Association.* Also, Ray E. Helfer and H. Kempe, *Child Abuse and Neglect. The Family and the Community.* Ballinger, Cambridge, Mass. 1976.

[4] Report of informal consultations among international non-governmental organizations on The Draft Convention on the Rights of the Child. Defence for Children International, Geneva. 1983, p. 10. See Art 8 bis. for definition of child abuse.

[5] In: Bourne and Newberger, *The Medicalization and Legalization of Child Abuse,* p. 701.

[6] In: Bernard Dickens, Legal Responses to Child Abuse. *Revue Canadienne de Droit Familiale.* Vol 1. 1978. Canadian Journal of Family Law.

[7] H.D.A. Freeman. *The Rights and Wrongs of Children.* 1983. France Pinter (Publisher London and Dover N.H. Pp. 111–115.

[8] Such as: Convention No. 138 (1973) on Minimum Age for Admission to Employment.
Convention on Slavery (1926) and Protocol
Convention on Suppression of Trafficking in Prostitution (1949)
Convention on Abolishment of Slavery, the Slave Trade and Institutions and Practice similar to Slavery (1956).
National Laws: Dowry Prohibition Act 1980 (Bangladesh)
Suppression of Immoral Traffic in Women and Girls, India, 1956.

[9] Shippen L Page. *The law, the lawyer, and medical aspects of child abuse.* See also, Douglas Besharov, Protecting Abused and Neglected Children. Can Law Help Social Work? *Child Abuse and Neglect* 7: 421–434 (1983).

[10] The 1974 Federal Child Abuse Prevention and Treatment Act. (Public Law 93–247). 42nd Cong. S85101 et seq. 88 Stat.7.

[11] B. Gil. *Violence against children.* Cambridge. Mass. Harvard University Press 1970.

[12] See the Field-Cisher Report into the Care and Supervision Provided in Relation to Maria Colwell, London, Her Majesty's Stationery Office, 1974.

[13] Latifa Akanda and Ishrat Shamim. Women and Violence. A comparative study of rural and urban violence on women in Bangladesh, 1984, Women for women. Elephant Road. Dakha. Bangladesh.

[14] See, Shippen Page, *The law, the lawyer and medical aspects of child abuse.* op. cit.

[15] Shropshire County Council. *Report of the Working Party of Social Services Committee Inquiry into the Circumstances Surrounding the Death of Graham Bagnall and the Role of the County Council's Social Services,* Shrewsbury, Shropshire CC. 1973.

[16] The Blom-Cooper Inquiry into the Death of Jasmine Bedford.

[17] Amrit Srinivasan. *Temple prostitution and community reform — the Devadasi case.* Paper delivered at the 2nd Asian Conference on Women and the Household. New Delhi, 1985. Indian Association for Women's Studies.

[18] Goldstein, Freud and Solnit. *Beyond the Best Interests of the Child.* New York, Free Press, 1979 (revised ed. Originally published 1973).

[19] See, F. Field, *Fair Shares for Families. The Need for a Family Impact Statement,* London, Study Commission on the Family, 1980 (p. 6. et seq.).

CHILD ABUSE AND NEGLECT: ALTERNATIVE APPROACHES

Jaap E. Doek*

Over the last 20 years the problem of the battered child has not suffered from lack of attention. On the contrary, endless numbers of books and articles have been written about the causes and consequences of child abuse and about the many and diverse forms of help and treatment projects and programmes set up to deal with it. However, regardless of how much is said or written about the abused child, one condition is essential if we are to help the child: the outside world — the neighbours, the family, the doctors, the social workers, etc. — must be made aware that the child in question is indeed being abused, and this knowledge, in turn, must be used to bring help to the child. In other words, identification and reporting of cases of child abuse are essential if we are to know what kind of help will be most effective. Therefore, in this discourse, I shall first discuss customary, and then the alternative, approaches to the problem of identification and reporting. It must be remembered that identification and reporting have no real purpose in themselves unless they are directed towards bringing about the most effective help possible to not only the abused child but also the family of which it is a part.

The phrase "alternative approaches" should be understood to mean non-judicial approaches; I shall not, at each point, refer to judicial/non-judicial. My greatest emphasis will be placed upon our experiences in the Netherlands and, where possible, a few references will be made to experiences in other countries.

IDENTIFICATION AND REPORTING

Reporting laws/legalizing the reporting of child abuse

To ensure that instances of child abuse are as quickly and effectively handled as possible, Reporting Laws were introduced in the U.S.A. during the second half of the 1960s. They made it obligatory for those, such as paediatricians, family doctors, nurses, social workers, etc., whose professional roles brought them into contact with possible cases of child abuse to report each case (or strong suspicion) of child abuse as defined by the law. This obligation in the course of the years not only resulted in an expansion of the definition of what constituted child abuse, but also increased the number of people who were required by law to report it. In some states every person is considered bound by law to report a case of child abuse.

It is not necessary at this point to go into the content and application of the Reporting Laws. They are referred to only as a well-known example of the judicial approach to identification and reporting of cases of child abuse. The United States example was followed by most of the provinces of Canada during the 1970s[1]. Another example of the judicial approach can be found in France.

---

* Professor, Faculteit der Rechtsgeleerdheid, Vrije Universiteit, Postbus 7161, 1007 MC Amsterdam, The Netherlands

One of the greatest hindrances to fast and effective reporting by doctors is the possible violation of professional confidentiality, which is itself punishable by law in many countries, including France. Until 1971, under Act 378 of the Penal Code, each violation of confidentiality was considered an offence; upholding professional confidentiality was strictly observed[2]. However, the law of June 15, 1971 revised Article 378 and since then doctors and all others bound by the code of confidentiality have been permitted to report to medical or administrative authorities any cases of abuse of children under the age of 15 they encounter in their practice. They are not required to report, or to appear as witnesses in judicial procedures.

In spite of this change in the law, Xuereb (see note) has noted that France and a number of other countries should re-examine their systems: "c'est le faible pourcentage de cas d'enfants maltraités signalés a la justice". In short, being free to report cases of child abuse voluntarily does not lead to quick and effective identification. The sad fact is that many children do not at all, or only too late, receive the help they need and to which they are entitled. From this we can draw the conclusion that compulsory reporting laws, such as those in the U.S.A., are indeed necessary. However, we should also look at the negative aspects of such laws:

(i) The reporting laws presume a "legal" approach to the problem of child abuse. I believe that this presumption is reinforced, particularly in the U.S., by requiring proof that the abuse occurred; this proof plays a decisive role in the judicial procedure aimed at protecting the child. It is obvious that this proof is critical in *criminal* proceedings, which may lead to the sentencing of the perpetrator, but why is it required in child protection procedures? The result is a very impersonal and formalized course of action controlled by formal regulations, which can further damage the already abused child and in no small measure needlessly invade the privacy of the whole family. Above all, it means that the legislation and legal decisions play a very important, probably decisive, role in shaping the approach to child abuse and neglect, determining the allocation of resources to this field[3].

(ii) The Reporting Laws and the associated Child Abuse Prevention and Treatment Act of 1974 can give the false impression that child abuse is being dealt with positively and effectively. Edward Zigler has pointed out that such laws "do little more than give us the false sense of security that something meaningful has been done, thus interfering with our mounting truly effective measures"[4].

(iii) There is little need for reporting laws particularly in countries where there are adequate organizations such as child protection services, welfare agencies and medical services that are alert to child abuse. Even without reporting laws, instances of child abuse can still be reported. This seems to be the case in England[5], but I doubt it[6]. If we look closely at what is happening in Europe it will be seen that many of the Western European countries, in spite of the number of child protection services, welfare agencies and medical services (for example, France, Belgium, the Federal Republic of Germany, the Scandinavian countries, Switzerland and the Netherlands) report very few cases of child abuse, not to speak of being able to present reasonably reliable statistical information on a national level as is done in the U.S.A. The conclusion must be that a legal process, based on reporting laws, has a number of shortcomings as means of encouraging the identification of cases of child abuse, but that for countries to have no reporting laws to compel them to deal with the problem leaves much to be desired.

I shall now present an alternative approach developed in the Netherlands to deal with the identification and reporting of cases of child abuse.

THE DUTCH REPORTING SYSTEM: THE CONFIDENTIAL DOCTOR BUREAU (CDB)

The origins of the CDB system[7]

At the end of the 1960s the press, radio and television in the Netherlands began to attract the attention of the public to child abuse. The Minister of Social Affairs and Public Health established a National Working Party on Child Abuse to devise a method by which, in particular, doctors who know that they are dealing with a case of child abuse should not have to keep it secret on grounds of professional confidentiality, but should be able to make it known to helping or judicial authorities. The working party proposed the establishment of four places in the Netherlands where "confidential doctors" would be designated as those with whom cases of child abuse could be discussed and reported. The object was to facilitate the reporting of cases of child abuse and to begin as quickly as possible the most suitable management of the child and the family. Also, it was intended as a means of making more information available about child abuse in the Netherlands.

The tasks of the confidential doctors were specified as follows:

(i) To advise anyone (not only a doctor) who reports a case of child abuse as to the best and most effective approach for that particular situation. If it seems necessary, the confidential doctor can take charge of the whole matter, when it is clear that the reporter cannot do so. Confidentiality is safeguarded because the notifier can get expert advice without going to the police or other (judicial) authorities. For doctors, the system is attractive because they can discuss the problem with a colleague (the confidential doctor is a paediatrician or a general practitioner) without violating professional confidentiality. Confidentiality is further assured by the regulation which states that only the confidential doctor may know the name of the reporter and that he may not divulge it to others (parents, child, police, protective services). If it becomes urgently necessary, for one reason or another, that someone else be told the name, it can be done only with the notifier's consent.

(ii) To collect information not only for the expansion of knowledge or to stimulate scientific research but also — and most important — to permit immediate action in cases of recidivism in a family.

(iii) To provide "after-care", which means that the confidential doctor sees to it that the treatment plan he has advised is implemented. He does this by checking with the notifier or the service or agency that has taken responsibility for the case; this after-care includes, if necessary, additional advice and adjustment of the treatment plan.

Since the first four confidential doctors were appointed in January 1972, the work has grown to the point that there are now 10 bureaus. They are organized as follows:

—one part-time paediatrician or general practitioner who maintains his private practice and devotes an average of eight hours a week, serving as the expert with the final responsibility for the activities of the bureau. There is also a deputy confidential doctor.
—one coordinator responsible for the administrative aspects of the work, i.e., first intake of telephone calls referring cases, registration, and organization of the after-care.
—one or more social workers who do the necessary checking and investigating of the reported cases and who also sometimes have direct contact with the services or agencies when there is a change of treatment.

The activities of the confidential doctor bureaus (CDB)

(i) The provision of advice

Since 1972 it has become apparent that the confidential doctors were sometimes notified of cases of child abuse for reasons other than to get advice about further treatment. The reports or notifications may be differentiated as follows:

—notification/referrals for registration purposes only (the notifier does not need advice) (group 1);
—notification for advice and consultation (group 2)
—notification with the request that the case be taken over, which means that the bureau is to refer the case to the most appropriate agency or service for treatment (group 3).

Before going further into these three forms of "notification", it should be pointed out that the last group has become, by far, the most important, accounting for more than 70% of the reported cases. This is a very sharp deviation from the original intent, which was simply to create a place for discussion and advice (group 2); see also Appendix 4.

Notification for registration purposes only (group 1) comes from organizations or persons who have themselves dealt with the matter or have referred it to the most appropriate health or welfare agency. All the confidential doctor does is to register the information provided. From this information, he can tell whether and when recidivism occurs.

Although notification for registration purposes serves to widen knowledge and prevent recidivism, one has the impression that the confidential doctor receives much less in this category than he should. Furthermore, the information reported is very limited; often, little is reported regarding the nature of the abuse, the help offered or the organizations involved. Thus, knowledge is not greatly expanded by these summary notifications for registration only. The voluntary nature of the notification to a confidential doctor is apparently the cause of these shortcomings. The confidential doctor's role here is a clearly passive, recording one.

Notification with a request for advice or consultation (group 2) accords fully with the confidential doctor's primary task. We are concerned here with reports from persons or bodies who themselves have facilities for offering or providing

133

(by referral) treatment or assistance but need consultation or want advice as to the most effective approach, which organizations should be involved, or the consequences of certain actions (e.g., involving the police). The confidential doctor's work in this case is as an active advisor. What this advice amounts to cannot be explained simply. It depends on the applicant's queries and the nature of the case; it may vary from confirming that a method already adopted is correct (with the advice being to continue), to urgently advising that the matter be referred to others, or even to leaving the case with the confidential doctor himself. It is clear that collecting data will be more successful with this form of notification than with notifications purely for recording purposes for no other reason than that the confidential doctor must have as much information as possible in order to give effective advice. In such cases, follow-up, i.e., information as to whether or not the advice was carried out, is of particular importance.

Notification with a request for referral (group 3) comes from that group of notifiers who, while bringing cases of child abuse to the confidential doctor's notice, wish to take it no further than that. The reason may be that they have no means of contributing towards further action or that they do not wish to harm an existing relationship with the family or the parents. The group includes, in particular, members of the family, neighbours, friends and also doctors and professional or voluntary workers who have contact with the family.

When this form of notification is made, the confidential doctor will himself have to set a treatment plan in motion. In many cases, the information will be too brief or too vague to undertake anything concrete. It is a firm rule with all bureaus that the family doctor or school doctor is the first to be approached. If necessary, the family doctor's identity is established. In this way, a check is made to determine whether the report should lead to certain steps and, if so, whether the family doctor or school doctor may be prepared to help. In other words, it is a matter not merely of checking the notification (i.e., whether it is at all likely or there are serious grounds for suspecting that child abuse occurred, as the neighbour or family member alleges) but also of finding a starting point for treatment. It is sometimes possible to refer the parents via the family or school doctor to a suitable welfare organization. This "medical" referral is the least threatening and the least stigmatizing (who is not at one time or another referred by his family doctor to an expert or a specialist?).

For further treatment, the confidential doctor may, if necessary, involve other organizations. Preference will then be given to those who have already had contact with the family or parents. To obtain this information, it is sometimes necessary to do some detective work. The activities of the confidential doctor after a notification with a request for referral clearly go further than the original working party's report anticipated. It is certainly more than a relatively passive advisory function. The confidential doctor is forced to initiate treatment himself when the notifier drops out. He must make and maintain contact with the treating organizations and sometimes with the family too.

It could be said that the confidential doctor takes the initiative and becomes the attendant on the case, i.e., he takes the first steps and makes the first contacts but then passes further treatment on to others as quickly as possible.

To be able to play this initiating role, the confidential doctor will have to obtain as much information as possible from an agency such as the Child Care and Protection Board. An *ad hoc* team is also usually formed, consisting of the confidential doctor and his staff and the staff of the organizations that are already, or should be, involved with the case.

All of these activities generally take place without the parents being aware of them. They begin to take notice only when a social worker or another welfare worker contacts them. There are some differences in practice on this point. Some confidential doctors spend little time searching for welfare organizations whose members might well be prepared to contact the family. Rather, the confidential doctors themselves approach the family fairly rapidly in order to assess the situation at first hand and to motivate the parents to accept help from others. However, most confidential doctors usually prefer to avoid this direct contact. They tend to observe the original intent, which was that the confidential doctor was to act only as advisor to the person reporting.

(ii) Organizational after-care

The confidential doctor is appointed not only to mount the most suitable assistance in cases of child abuse by giving advice or initiating some form of help but also to make sure that the assistance given is maintained and not withdrawn prematurely. For this, the confidential doctor follows up, by telephone or letter, after a certain period, which varies, according to the nature of the problem, from three to six months. The purposes of this contact are:

(1) to make certain that treatment is not becoming bogged down;
(2) to advise on any interim adjustment to the treatment plan;
(3) if necessary, to ensure that treatment is duly transferred to another body;
(4) to advise whether assistance should be ended; and,
(5) to keep the situation of other children in the family under scrutiny.

Such after-care is planned when a welfare worker is involved. The information requested is generally readily supplied. However, it is extremely summary and often limited to a statement of the welfare worker that the family is still receiving treatment or that the case is closed. Sometimes when problems arise the welfare worker will himself contact the confidential doctor. Some confidential doctors take such after-care very seriously and translate it in practice to a personal responsibility for the progress of the case. Indeed, if a welfare worker involved by the confidential doctor ceases his work because he considers it no longer necessary, some confidential doctors like to check that this decision is correct and will initiate further assistance if necessary. The welfare worker is, of course, likely to see this as an expression of no confidence. Other confidential doctors stop at less far-reaching after-care, taking the view that the welfare worker has his own responsibilities. These differences apart, organizational after-care has remained an underdeveloped aspect of the confidential doctor's task. This is probably due largely to its open-ended character. The welfare worker involved by the doctor is not obliged to provide any information at all. He is free to react as he wishes to an amicable request from the doctor to keep him informed about the state of affairs. The confidential doctor may feel uncomfortable if asked to monitor something without having explicit statutory powers to do so.

(iii) The gathering of data

The outcome of this task of the confidential doctor is an annual report containing a great deal of information on such items as the ages of child and perpetrator, their sex, the position of the child in the family, parents' occupation and social class, and the nature of the abuse. The reports for the years up to and including 1980 have now been published. Regrettably, there is no indication that they have so far given any impetus to intensive scientific research. In brief, one could say that we now know a great deal about child abuse, but little about the effects of the treatment applied.

The results: improved detection and treatment

First: since 1972 about 15 000 abused children have been brought to the attention of the confidential doctors (see Appendix 1) and a great deal of information has been collected (e.g., age, type of abuse/neglect, sources from which the reports came: see Appendices 2, 3, 4).

Thanks to the work of the Bureaus these abused children have received the help and treatment they needed when it was needed (before 1972 they did not receive this additional attention). This is the most important result of the positive actions of the confidential doctor. Precisely because of the intervention of the confidential doctor and his staff, account has been taken of the treatment of abused children and of the associated risks to the child (the danger of repetition, for example). The organizational after-care by the confidential doctor has meant that treatment continued in the most suitable way as long as it was necessary (premature termination was countered; the risk of recidivism was pointed out, etc). In short, the outcome has been clearly beneficial for the maltreated child.

Another important result relates to provisions for assistance and treatment. Through the work of the confidential doctor, organizations which before 1972 did not, or did not wish to, recognize child abuse have been confronted with it. The confidential doctor's simple question "would you help a maltreated child *and* his parents who have been reported to me?" forced them to think about child abuse (denial was no longer possible), about the methods of giving help up to this point, and about their prejudices and emotions towards abusive parents. In this way, various organizations concerned with social work and health care generally have begun to assist maltreated children in more conscious and expeditious ways. Also, their skill in the early detection of child abuse has improved. They have come to pay more attention to the possibility of the occurrence of child abuse and to know how to provide suitable assistance via the confidential doctor. Certain organizations take very special notice of maltreated children and their parents, others are beginning to do so. The effects outlined above have been further strengthened by the advice that the confidential doctors regularly give to the organizations with which they work in their areas.

In summary, it may be said that the confidential doctor's work has promoted and improved the detection and treatment of maltreated children by their use of the existing facilities.

This is an important structural gain in that the maltreated children and their parents are no longer unnecessarily isolated by institutions specially entrusted with the care of maltreated children. There children and their parents enter by the same door as parents and children with other problems. No institutionalized distinction is drawn between abuse and other problems of child-rearing, other than, of course, treatment by the assisting organization.

These results have been achieved without extensive legislation or incisive organizational changes and may be regarded as positive, though it should not be inferred that every maltreated child in the Netherlands receives optimal assistance. It must be remembered that the confidential doctor is involved on a voluntary basis. Many maltreated children never come to his attention. They are detected either too late or not at all because there still are persons in a position to provide aid who do not see, or do not wish to see, the problem. In brief, much still has to be done in improving detection, involving the confidential doctor, and stimulating general awareness.

The confidential doctor system: a non-judicial approach

As has already been pointed out, the use of the confidential doctor constitutes a reporting system that is, to the best of my knowledge, the only systematically applied model of a non-judicial approach to the detection and treatment of cases of child abuse. There is no requirement to report the system is based completely upon the voluntary cooperation of professionals working in the field of child abuse and of the entire population. Thus, it has evolved as a totally informal reporting system or model; there is not the slightest legal obligation upon the bureaus to carry out their work.

I do not say that these aspects are favourable. On the contrary, I consider them to be the weak links in the system (see the next section). However, what I consider most important, in addition to the non-stigmatizing, integrating effects of using services and agencies that are not specifically designated for child abuse, is that the system allows the best use of non-coercive, voluntary facilities; only as a last resort is the use of the courts or police considered. This does *not* mean that criminal prosecution and sentencing has no place, or that the Children's Court judge is not brought in to take protective measures. What is true, however, is that judicial intervention is sought only after very careful consideration and when it is absolutely necessary; it is not sought automatically. In a way, the role of the confidential doctor may be viewed as a diversionary one.

The Netherlands figures (see Appendix 5) are very revealing. If we bear in mind that those instances of child abuse that are reported to the Confidential Doctors Bureau are, in greatest measure, the most serious forms of child abuse, the percentage of cases that must ultimately be remanded to the court for prosecution or to the Children's Court judge for protective measures is quite small.

The confidential doctor system: a European reporting system?

The Netherlands reporting system is being followed, albeit on a very small scale, in Belgium[8] and it is attracting attention in the Federal Republic of Germany[9]; quite recently (June 10, 1985) the representatives of the Federal Republic took the initiative in the European Parliament (in the Commission for Youth, Culture, Education, Information and Sport) to ask that specific guidelines be established to coordinate action against child abuse. The proposal as it is at present worded, recommends, among other things, the following:

—"in Zuzammenarbeit mit der Europaischen Gemeinschaft und den Nieder-

landen in einem Modell-versuch erproben ob das ubertragen werden kann".
Also, there is some discussion about "eine Melde — und Beratungs stelle".

In any event, it would be interesting to exchange ideas about the possibility as well as the desirability of having a European reporting system based on the Netherlands model. I am reminded of the Recommendations of the Council of Europe in 1969 and 1979[10] concerning the protection of children against maltreatment. The 1979 Recommendations included an invitation to the member states, "with a view to ensuring in the most effective way, prevention, detection and management of cases of child abuse," to improve the organization of the child welfare system.

Obviously the Netherlands model could not be expected to function unaltered at the European level, because there are too many national differences. But I feel very strongly that it could serve as a basis for further consideration if the countries concerned were to agree on the aim of a single reporting system which would:

—be clearly based upon a medical-social-community model in which all cases of child abuse could be reported either for registration, advice and consultation or for further treatment;
—at the same time make use of the existing facilities for the protection and treatment of cases of child abuse;
—ensure that the maltreated child, as soon as a report is received, receives the most suitable treatment for as long as necessary and that the treatment is monitored and adjusted as needed (organizational after-care);
—mobilize the existing helping facilities on a voluntary basis and also function in a diversionary capacity.

From the Netherlands experience I would warn anyone wishing to introduce the reporting system that they do so with certain stipulations. From its inception, and certainly within five years of setting up the system, particular attention should be paid to the following:

(i) There should be good control over the qualifications of the staff of the Bureau and its co-workers, with special attention to maintaining professional confidentiality; and also over the provisions for organizational after-care, that is, the follow-up of those children sent on to services or agencies for child protection, welfare or treatment.
(ii) There should be a regulation to protect the privacy of the families (parents, children) who are reported to the Bureau; it must be kept in mind that sometimes the report may be unjustified.
(iii) The reporting system should be voluntary, but for certain groups of people (professionals) reporting should be made compulsory and the obligation to report should be backed up by the law.

Finally, it is most important that any country that proposes to establish such a system has at least a reasonably well developed, preferably a highly developed, network of welfare services, child protection agencies and medical treatment facilities.

Notes

[1] See B. Chisholm, *Question of social policy — a Canadian perspective*. In: *Family violence, an international and interdisciplinary study*, p. 318–329, edited by J.M. Echelaar and S.N. Katz (Butterworths, Toronto 1978) who reports that nine of the twelve provinces of Canada have legislation making reporting of child abuse mandatory.

[2] The classical formula, which has been used in this respect repeatedly, amongst others in a decision of the Cour de Cassation, chambre criminelle, on 22 Dec 1966, reads as follows: "L'obligation au secret professionel établie et sanctionnée par l'article 378 du Code Pénal pour assurer le confiance nécessaire à l'exercice de certains professions, s'impose au médecin comme un devoir d'état. Elle est générale et absolue et il n'appartient à personne de l'en affranchir". For more information see, e.g., J.C. Xuereb, Les fondements et la pratique de l'intervention judiciare. In: *L'Enfant maltraité* (pp. 145–167), par P. Straus et M. Manciaux (Editions Fleurus, Paris, 1982).

[3] See E.H. Newberger and R. Bourne, *The medicalization and legalization of child abuse*. In: *Critical perspectives on child abuse*, by the same authors (Lexington Books, Massachusetts, 1979) pp. 139–157.

[4] See E. Zigler, *Controlling child abuse in America: an effort doomed to failure?* In: *Critical perspectives on child abuse* (see note 3) pp. 171–215.

[5] J. Stark, *The battered child — does Britain need a reporting law? Public Law, 1969*, pp. 48–63. "Britain does not need a reporting law to designate agencies to receive and initiate actions on behalf of the child. Both local authorities' children's departments and the NSPCC have powers wide enough for action..."

[6] See also J.G. Hall and B.H. Mitchell, *The role of the law in protecting the child; a critique of the English system*. In: *Child Abuse and Neglect, 6* (1982) pp. 63–69.

[7] See for more information about the background of the creation of the Confidential Doctors' Bureaus and the legal context in which they are working: J.E. Doek, *Child abuse in the Netherlands: the medical referee*, Chicago, *Kent Law Review 54*(3) (1978) pp. 785–826; and also J.E. Doek and S. Slagter, *Child care and protection in the Netherlands* (Amsterdam 1979, Stichting voor het Kind).

[8] A confidential doctor bureau was established in Antwerp in 1979, the so-called Vertrouwenarts centrum. This centre works along the same lines as the Dutch system. See: R. Clara, *The confidential doctor centre: a medical model for an effective attack on child abuse*. In: *Scientific investigation in Belgium with regard to child abuse*, pp. 43–75, (published by the Belgian organization against child abuse: Child and Violence, Antwerp, 1983). See also R. Clara c.s. *Vertrouwensartscentrum-Antwerpen* (Confidential doctors centre of Antwerp), *Child abuse and neglect, 6* (1982), pp. 233–237.

[9] See A.J. Koers, *Kindesmishandelung und Kinderschutz in den Niederlanden*. In: *Gewalt gegen Kinder*, H. Bast c.s. (Arbeitsgruppe Kinderschutz), pp. 278–313 (Rowohlt Verlag 1975).

[10] Recommendation 561 (1969) adopted by the Assembly on September 30, 1969 and Recommendation No. R(79) 17 of the Committee of Ministers to Member States (adopted by the Committee on September 13, 1979).

Appendix 1 Number of reports to the Confidential Doctors Bureaus 1972–1980.

Source: Annual Reports of CDB

Year	Number of Centres	Total number of reports	Concerning child abuse	Not concerning child abuse	Number of re- ported children
1972	4	420	430	45	430
1973	4	628	628	—	628
1974	6	981	823	158	823
1975	7	1071	815	255	815
1976	9	1289	899	390	896
1977	10	1729	1317	412	1249
1978	10	2796	2075	721	1975
1979	10	3086	2378	708	2378
1980	10	3029	2228	801	2228
1983*	10	3300	2275	—	2275

* preliminary figures

140

Appendix 2 Proportional figures of the types of abuse reported to confidential doctor bureaus (100% = the total amount of reported types). It is possible that more than one type of abuse is reported about one child.

Source: Calculations are based on the figures of the annual reports of the confidential doctor bureaus.

Nature of maltreatment		Year 1972	1973	1974	1975	1976	1977	1978	1980
Physical abuse	1.	38.1	24.7	23.9	21.8	23.4	18.7	15.6	19.5
	2.	17.2	16.2	19.9	20.5	16.5	16.5	16.4	16.1
	3.	8.6	12.9	11.2	12.9	11.4	12.5	12.2	10.9
	4.	1.2	2.1	1.8	1.3	0.4	1.0	0.6	—
Total		65.1	55.9	56.7	56.5	51.7	48.6	44.7	46.5
Physical neglect	1.	—	8.4	11.8	12.3	9.4	8.6	11.5	9.0
	2.	—	4.1	3.2	6.3	4.5	6.7	7.6	3.9
	3.	—	0.7	0.9	1.6	1.7	2.2	2.8	1.5
	4.	—	0.3	0.0	0.0	0.0	0.0	0.2	—
Total		—	13.5	15.9	20.3	15.6	17.6	22.2	14.4
Emotional abuse	1.	5.8	4.8	7.7	6.1	10.1	9.0	10.3	12.9
	2.	7.7	4.8	6.2	6.4	8.6	10.2	9.7	12.9
	3.	4.2	3.5	2.3	3.7	5.4	7.5	8.1	6.0
	4.	0.7	0.3	0.4	0.4	0.4	1.4	0.7	—
Total		18.4	13.5	16.6	16.6	24.4	28.0	28.8	31.8
Sexual abuse	1.	—	0.7	0.7	0.4	0.5	0.5	0.3	0.2
	2.	—	1.7	1.3	0.9	0.6	1.3	0.6	1.8
	3.	—	2.0	1.0	1.9	1.9	1.6	1.4	2.1
	4.	—	0.4	0.1	0.2	0.2	0.1	0.3	—
Total		—	4.8	3.1	3.3	3.2	3.6	2.6	7.7
Both physical and emotional abuse		11.8	—	—	—	—	—	—	—
Unknown		4.7	12.3	7.8	3.3	5.0	2.1	1.7	3.05
TOTAL		100.0	100.0	100.0	100.0	99.9	99.9	100.0	100.0

Explanation
1. = age group 0–5 years
2. = age group 6–11 years
3. = age group 12–17 years
4. = age group above 18 years.
The figures behind 'Total' are not always exactly the sum of the column owing to rounding in decimals.

Appendix 3 Proportional figures of reports concerning child abuse from reporters.

Source: Annual reports of Confidential Doctor Bureaus.

Professional workers		1972	1973	1974	1975	1976	1977	1978	1980	1983*
Doctors	m	35.8	26.3	28.3	29.8	31.9	27.4	22.1	18.4	17.3
Child health centres		4.4	8.4	4.4	2.7	4.0	1.8	1.7	2.9	2.5
District-nursing/family care		3.3	1.4	2.3	1.3	2.3	2.4	1.9	2.9	3.0
Child Care and Protection Board	j	10.2	9.1	9.8	8.5	6.8	7.2	5.9	3.4	3.3
Institutions for child protection		0.7	1.8	1.5	1.5	1.7	2.7	2.0	1.2	1.0
Police		4.9	4.5	4.1	6.3	8.8	8.3	6.1	7.5	8.2
Social work/welfare service		4.7	4.1	4.4	5.2	3.7	7.4	7.1	4.8	9.0
Total of professional workers		64.0	55.6	54.8	55.3	59.2	57.2	46.8	40.1	77.3
Educators and others who come into contact with children professionally										
Teachers		6.5	4.6	3.3	5.8	6.1	7.1	8.0	7.7	10.0
Day nursery/day care centres		0.5	0.3	2.3	0.6	0.1	0.5	1.0	1.3	0.5
Total		7.0	4.9	5.6	6.4	6.2	7.6	9.0	9.0	10.5
Parents and children		5.3	7.5	6.0	8.0	4.8	7.5	6.8	6.6	8.0
Relatives, neighbours, friends and acquaintances		16.5	21.8	23.6	18.4	18.2	18.5	25.5	27.2	28.6
Unknown/anonymous/others		7.2	10.2	10.0	11.9	11.6	9.2	11.9	16.0	8.5
Total		100.0	100.0	100.0	100.0	100.0	100.0	100.0	100.0	100.0
Total number of reports		430	628	823	815	899	1317	2075	2228	

Explanation:
m = medical   j = judicial   *preliminary figures.

142

Appendix 4 Purpose of reports and following action of Centres of Confidential Doctors.

Source: Annual Reports of Confidential Doctor Bureaus.

Reporter's request to Bureau of C.D.	1972	1973	1974	1975	1976	1977	1978	1980	1983*
Purely for registration	—	19.4	21.0	12.8	12.9	11.2	8.4	5.6	7.5
With request for advice	—	28.5	17.6	8.2	11.3	16.7	17.5	9.3	13.5
Further treatment left to C.D.	—	50.8	61.4	78.2	74.7	71.6	73.5	85.1	79.0
Unknown	—	1.3	—	0.9	1.1	0.5	0.5	—	—
Total number of reports	430	628	823	815	899	1317	2075	2228	

Nature of activities of the C.D.	1972	1973	1974	1975	1976	1977	1978	1980	1983
Advising	—	19.3	12.5	10.1	13.7	9.3	10.4	16.8	16.83
Taking initiatives	—	56.6	68.2	76.5	72.7	80.6	83.4	68.0	74.8
Purely registering	—	24.1	19.3	13.4	13.6	9.7	6.2	15.2	10.38
Total number of reports	430	628	823	815	899	1317	2075	2228	—

* Preliminary figures.

Appendix 5 Judicial intervention in child abuse cases reported to the Confidential Doctor Bureaus

Source: Annual reports of the Confidential Doctor Bureau

A Child protective measures by juvenile judge/court after the case was reported to CDB.
1.

	number	percentage
1973	60	9,9
1974	69	8,4
1975	72	8,8
1976	100	11,1
1977	146	11,1
1978	249	12,0
1979	240	13,7
1980	245	14,9

B Criminal prosecution of the perpetrators in cases reported to the CDB.

	total number of perpetrators	number of prosecuted	percentage
1973	606	8	1,3
1974	823	26	3,2
1975	815	24	1,7
1976	794	17	2,1
1977	1005	21	2,1
1978	1695	24	1,4
1979*	—	—	—
1980*	—	—	—

* no figures available.

DISCUSSION

Gellhorn: Thank you very much Mrs Owen and Dr Doek. You have introduced a number of provocative subjects for comment. I hope we will have some discussion about Mrs Owen's suggestion for an ombudsman for children, the breadth of the mandatory reporting that she suggested, the screening of babysitters — in the US it would be quite a job to screen all of our babysitters, but perhaps it is something that is indicated. I think that in this sophisticated audience many already know the story that I just learned about as I was preparing to come to this meeting. In 1874 in New York there was the case of the child, Mary Ellen, who was discovered by the nurse, Eda Wheeler, chained to a bed-post, as she had been for some time, under conditions of starvation and abuse. Eda Wheeler then attempted to provide some protection of this child but found there were no means of protecting the child in New York. So she turned to the Society for the Prevention of Cruelty to Animals and had the child sent to the Society on the basis that humans were also animals. And from there, then developed, in 1875, the first Society for the Prevention of Cruelty to Children.

Clara: I am not going to speak about the confidential doctor centre but I would stress Mrs Owen's point that not enough money is spent for children. I believe on the basis of studies made last year that less and less money is given for children. We don't live in the year of the child, we live in the year of the old people, because more and more money is going to the old, who are much more politically influential than the young people and their parents. We see in Scientific American of December 1984 that in the last 10 or 15 years in the United States the money spent for children was diminished by 50% while what was spent for old people rose dramatically. So I believe that not only for medical care and for social care, but also for education, more young persons should be given subventions, because more people are living in poverty.

Gellhorn: I certainly wish to second your comment, Dr Clara, noting that particularly in our country we old people have a strong and very effective lobby. There is only one children's defence fund in our country that is effective and that is principally for children in poverty. It does very well but cannot be compared to the old folk's lobby.

Morrow: I would like to ask Dr Doek several questions. First, he quite impressed upon us that the confidential doctor system prevents stigmatization. Now, is it acknowledged, or has concern been expressed, in the Netherlands that although it may not stigmatize in one respect, perhaps by using the medical model it medicalizes the problem? One might ask, for example, why not a confidential nurse or a confidential teacher or even a confidential lawyer to be the focus for these reports and whether using a doctor assists society in blaming the victims of child violence, which of course are not just the children but the parents as well. Can I ask a second question — issues not only of professional confidentiality arise, and I was interested to hear him refer to this — but surely also issues of professional accountability and responsibility. To what extent do the other professions involved — social workers, nurses, school doctors, etc. — take to

145

what appears to be quite an active directive role on the part of the confidential doctor? Do they actually respond to this confidential doctor telling them what to do? I know in my own country the general practitioner's or paediatrician's role as the leader of the health care team is in question in this respect. Finally, could I ask whether the confidential doctor has any input into developing preventive interventions, and does he have to account for the work of his bureau in, for example, an annual report, which might serve to look at possible preventive interventions?

Doek: The simple reason for having a paediatrician or a general practitioner has to do with our law on professional confidentiality. The idea behind having a doctor is that as long as you discuss the case with that doctor — general practitioner or paediatrician — you are within the circle of people bound by professional confidentiality, so you don't violate confidentiality. What is not discussed at all in that regard is what happens when the confidential doctor goes to a social worker and says he has had a case referred from the paediatrician from this or that hospital, asking him to set some treatment in motion, and asks whether the social worker is willing to join in trying to treat the case. This is, in my opinion, a violation of confidentiality, but it is a point which we in the Netherlands don't discuss, maybe on the basis of the philosophy that, if you don't discuss it, it doesn't exist.

The second point: I agree with you that the medical model, which appears to be the model for the confidential doctor bureau, is criticized in the Netherlands and for that reason I think the social worker's role within the bureau is important. There are indications that in the Netherlands we are moving more and more in the direction of a medical-social model, rather than a purely medical model. But there is a problem there: the professional accountability of the people involved. One of the weak spots of the system is that it is a voluntary system and you involve as a bureau outside social workers or protective workers in the child protective area; you do so on a voluntary basis. This means that you discuss the case, you make a treatment plan, you plan activities of different people, and you come back after three or six months to discuss the progress of the treatment of the parents and the child. There is in theory the possibility that the social worker whom, as a confidential doctor, you have involved does not report to you. It doesn't happen very often but it is a very weak spot. We rely on our voluntary system almost completely for the way the professionals keep their professional code; if they are involved in a case, and there is an agreement on reporting after three or six months, we take it that they do report. If they don't, there is no legal provision for forcing them to do it. The last point, involving preventive action: confidential doctors and their associated social workers give presentations to inform professionals and volunteers in the fields of welfare, child protection and health care about child abuse and neglect, which has some preventive effects, I think.

Gellhorn: Thank you, Dr Doek. Some time we should have a discussion on doctors' codes and what they mean or do not mean.

Owen: I should like to offer some comment on the very important problem of resources. First, I must emphasize that when governments make cuts in public services, such as child-care facilities and nursery schools, the immediate burden falls on women, although the consequential effect inevitably is on children. Secondly, it has to be recognized that, whereas women form a constituency, in the sense of being able to voice grievances, children do not. I was in Nairobi this summer for the NGO Forum for the end of the UN Decade for Women. Whenever we talked about violence, exploitation, prostitution, we were always conscious that millions of children were also caught up in these forms of abuse, and that ultimately it was children who suffered: the two themes are indissolubly related, but with the essential difference, as I have just mentioned, that the adult has, in principle at least, an opportunity to protest, not available to the child. That is why we need, perhaps, a children's ombudsman. In this respect, we have to acknowledge that UNICEF, in its child survival programme, has major achievements to its credit internationally. But it too has limited resources; more are needed if UNICEF is to extend its activities to include consideration of the quality of life of those children who survive. Finally, I wish to raise a matter I was discussing a short time ago with Dr Krugman. In developed countries, at any rate, should we not be thinking about how children who have been injured, battered, abused can be compensated through dispositions made by the courts, family or criminal, depending on the legislative system? I understand that in the USA a scheme, operative during the last few years, earmarks funds available either for the compensation of children who have suffered injury or abuse, or for the support of programmes to treat children and the families who have abused them. This question of compensation is, in my view, one which deserves consideration by this workshop.

Vesterdal: Professor Doek, as far as I heard, you said that in Europe there were no laws about reporting, but you haven't included Denmark in Europe. We have a law that anybody who sees a child or youngster below the age of 18 years who needs help from the social service has to report it, and it is emphasized that doctors also have to do it, despite the observance of professional secrecy; this includes child abuse and neglect, but the wording is very soft and borderline cases also can be included. It is not so bad for the families, the legal system is there. What we lack is more information to use the social system in the right way.

Belsey: Both speakers have given us a very good perspective and varying experiences on legislation and non-legislative approaches. Perhaps, however, they might devote a few minutes to comment not on the therapeutic or after-the-fact aspects, but on the role of legislation and non-legislative action in promotive and preventive aspects. We have heard yesterday and also this morning about this sort of background noise, this social climate of violence, of sexual exploitation. Richard Krugman showed an excellent photo of the subtle, and not so subtle, exploitation that serves as a background against which child abuse, neglect, sexual exploitation take place. What is the role of the approaches you have put forward at the level of prevention and promotion, going down to the question of schools, the question of school curriculum? What can and cannot be taught in schools *vis-à-vis* healthy parenthood and some of the problems that may arise in parenthood, in order to prepare adolescents so that they don't become abusing parents.

Doek: Just as an example. I happen to be President of the Dutch Society for the Prevention of Child Abuse. In my opinion such a national society on child abuse and neglect can do very important things in the preventive and health promotive areas. To give you an example of what we did as a national society, we developed a package of materials which can be used by teachers in the primary schools, for children between the ages of 6 and 12 years, and another package for those colleges where teachers and social workers are being trained. For primary-school teachers, for instance, there is a very well elaborated and thoughtful, step-by-step programme by which they can teach children, not what is child abuse, but how you deal with children if you are a parent, what is allowed and what is good, and what is bad about treating children. We have recently published a book with stories about child abuse; it was published together with guidelines for its use in classrooms in primary schools, but children also can read it, because the stories are simple, for children. So there are various ways of doing it. If you have such a national group of people who mainly consist of volunteers you can do many things in the area of prevention.

Owen: First, I think that governments should support the voluntary agencies that work for children. For example, in new areas of concern such as child sexual abuse, it is the voluntary agencies that have stepped in first, gathering information, undertaking research, creating public awareness and pioneering preventive programmes. Their responses, successes and failures need careful evaluation. Governments should support these voluntary initiatives, study their effectiveness, and provide resources for their expansion, continuity and monitoring.

Second, the role of public education and information in preventing child abuse cannot be over-emphasized. Research findings have suggested that the presentation of violence and sexual activities on film, television and video is connected with juvenile delinquency, drug usage and child abuse, especially sexual abuse. The law cannot effectively ban "snuff movies", child pornography and other "nasty" videos, but governments can promote educational campaigns directed at parents, teachers and the general public so that they are made aware of these dangers in society today and are thus informed sufficiently to take their own effective preventive action.

Third, we have to prepare today's children for tomorrow's responsible parenthood. The law can facilitate, rather than obstruct, the provision of family-planning information and services to adolescents so that unwanted babies (the most likely victims of child abuse) are not born. Also, parenthood education should not be limited to girls. Last year in Britain an interesting experiment was undertaken in a boys' detention centre. Boys of 13–15 years were instructed how to bathe, feed and care for a baby, using rubber dolls as models. The programme raised eyebrows in some circles but not for long. The logic is there. Those young boys will be fathers in a few years time. Their spell in detention will not have been wasted if they emerge with some idea of responsible parental behaviour. This is an example of how a voluntary initiative caught on and was taken up by the statutory services.

Diaz: I agree fully with Professor Doek that the first step towards doing anything for children who are abused and neglected and abandoned is to identify them.

We have just completed a photo-documentation work in Africa on this, and in one of the countries we found that the abused children are carted away by the police and put into jail or somewhere where they will never be seen at all. There is a lot of work to be done in changing the level of acceptance of society of the realities of child abuse and neglect. The trend in developing countries will be on the increase, and we have to think of ways by which we can create awareness through the mass media, through institutional channels, schools, churches, professional groups and through change agents, through interpersonal communication media.

With regard to the issue of law — I think the legal systems in developing countries don't work for these children because they are too complex where 75% of women are illiterate. Also we neglect common-law arrangements, which are more reconciliatory than the adversarial system, where the legal provisions protect the establishment rather than the poor and neglected. There is a need to develop this traditional system of dealing with children who are abused and neglected, as well as perhaps utilizing legal systems by means of legal aid which will reach slum areas and rural areas. Perhaps this forum could suggest that the United Nations declare a year, an international year, for abused and neglected children, just to dramatize this point, because the problem is increasing in a lot of developing countries where we are working.

Obikeze: I wish to more or less complement the last speaker on the issue of laws, with particular reference to labour laws. One of the previous speakers has said that child and labour laws in the developing countries do not work and should be thrown away. I think I agree. But what I need to call attention to is that part of the reason why these laws do not work lies in their *origin.* We need to look into how these laws came about in the first place to see why they cannot work.

Normally, laws should arise from and be rooted in the norms and value systems of a people. They should reflect what the people think to be proper ways of doing things. It is when such normative codes are synthesized into laws that they have every chance of being obeyed, that they have a chance of being accepted by the people. When laws are imposed on a society, irrespective of prevailing patterns of life, they risk being rejected or ignored. This has happened with regard to laws proposed by the International Labour Organization and other international organizations,when they were enacted without regard to prevailing socioeconomic patterns, the way each society concerned has been managing its economic and productive life. I feel I should call attention to this particular area to emphasize the need to carry out research into a people's lifestyle before making laws for them.

Gellhorn: I suppose there is no comment on that except that my reaction is that we must not call on research and more research, and not do anything in the meantime, which is a very great hazard. It is always so much easier to say we had better do some more research and in the meantime we do nothing for the child.

Krugman: I have two random comments, and if this morning's two speakers, Mrs Owen and Professor Doek, would like to comment I should be delighted. I want to thank both of them for their presentations, I thought they put the issue into perspective. One addition I would make — and I borrow from Ray Helfer again — is that at a conference in Arizona last year he issued a challenge to many of the judges and lawyers who were present. We were discussing sexual abuse and the statement was made that the legal system was not working for children. Ray drew the analogy to what happened in medicine about 50 years ago when there was no such thing as paediatrics. One approached children as an adult internist and one did a physical examination the way one was taught in medical school to examine an adult; one would first examine the head, then the ears, then the eyes, nose and throat, and proceed throughout in a very systematic, adult-oriented fashion. If one tried to do that with a child, particularly a very young child, the examination would be over after the ears, and one would have no further information because the child would be in tears and screaming, and all of the information one wanted would be lost. The challenge, basically, to the legal system is that we have a very adult-oriented system. It has been developed to respond to adult needs in criminal and civil matters. What we need is for good minds, such as the two we have down on the podium right now, to think about how you take an adult-oriented system of laws, civil and criminal, and make it work for children. That doesn't mean you throw out constitutions or that you throw out laws, but you look for creative ways to get the law to work for children. Now there are approaches that Mrs Owen mentioned about video-taping in the United States, and that is one approach. I think, in contrast to the comment that was made just a moment ago by the gentleman from UNICEF, that the law does not need to be adversarial; it can be used on behalf of children if one will think about how to use it. Courts can ask for more information. We try not to blame people in a civil court when we bring in an abuse case in the United States. We say it is not a matter of who did it, and blame; it as a matter of the child's safety. Is this child abused or not? If the answer is yes, the child is not safe; then the court needs more information. That information may involve psychological evaluation, psychiatric evaluation; it may involve a variety of things that will let the court act to place the child in a safe place and to order treatment. No blame, no fault. That is one point. The second point is that children don't vote, and we have to rely on children's defence funds and others. But I would hope that someone would try to enfranchise children by giving parents the same number of votes as the number of children they have. I don't think it can happen in our country at the moment but I would hope that in perhaps one of your countries or jurisdictions it might be tried. Now before everybody tells me what is wrong with that, I can assure you that I know no country where the vote is so valuable that this would interfere with family-planning efforts. I don't think that people will have 10 or 15 children just to get 10 or 15 votes. But I do think that, if children were enfranchized in this way, many parents when their children were over 12 or 14 would let them vote on certain initiatives. I know that two of my children would not vote the same as I do on a lot of issues and it is probably good for them to be able to represent themselves. I also suggest that this proposal would dramatically change budgetary priorities for local, state, and national governments, which might find that 40–50% of the population were more interested in social programmes and food than in guns; they might find the national priorities different. I should like somebody to pick up on that at least.

Doek: It was a long story and a long question. I will pick one — the last because it is not as crazy as you think, or maybe it is just that others told you that it is. The

150

problem is how to proceed — children don't vote and that it is a very important point in the whole issue of child protection and child care, child abuse, whatever. It has effects on the budget, on the way politicians make decisions.

Owen: What has been said points to the need for either a special government ministry for children or an ombudsman; that is to say, a central unit within government that can examine all the needs of children, at present handled in a fragmentary way by a number of different departments. In addition, I think that we have to use to the utmost the media — the press, television etc. — to publicize what the rights of children are and to remove from children themselves that fear of the law which equates it to a policeman who is going to take them away from home, put them before a court and send them away to detention. Children have to understand that the law is there to help and protect them. Indeed, they can even assist in bringing about changes in the law.

Countries might also consider developing a "children's parliament". It could provide opportunities for children to learn what their rights are and how to exercise them. Certainly there should be a national children's commission, and mature children could play an active role in it. I also think that all countries should establish children's legal centres, staffed possibly by volunteer lawyers, who could provide direct legal advice to children in trouble with the law, with police, with their schools, their families or employers. Lastly, we should be examining whether the arrangements in existing juvenile courts, particularly the adversarial system, really promote the welfare of the child and provide the appropriate setting for making crucial decisions affecting his or her future life. Scotland now has a non-adversarial system for deciding such matters. The adult-oriented court, its procedures and scenario, may not be in the child's best interests.

Gill: We seem to accent very much the poor in these deliberations but we know of instances of child abuse in even the richest families. Secondly, as paediatricians nowadays in the developed countries, we see parental systems that are sure to fail for children. I mean immature, isolated, ill-prepared and very young parents, whose children in the future are at greater risk.

REPORTS OF DISCUSSION GROUPS

GROUP A: Types of resources

Moderator: F. Reyes Romero
Secretary: M. Carballo

The group recognized that child abuse or maltreatment occurs in a variety of forms. In many parts of the world its manifestation is primarily societal; large numbers of children are affected, to the extent that the abuse becomes societal and is often confused with traditional or cultural phenomena. In developing countries this is being provoked and maintained through wars, poverty, ignorance and malnutrition, and millions of children are affected. The presentation ranges from chronic malnutrition (non-organic failure to thrive) to retarded growth and development as a result of exploitative child labour practices, and psychosocial injury due to protracted war conditions, into which children are being increasingly drawn.

This widespread and pervasive form of child abuse should not be obscured by the dramatic nature of other forms of child abuse, which are serious and involve child battering, but which affect fewer children and yet receive considerably more attention.

Societal child abuse provokes patterns of child mortality and chronic morbidity that account for the annual deaths of up to 200 per 1,000 live births in the countries affected. It is typical of many developing countries and is influenced by both international and national economic policies. The group felt that the efforts of all international and national bodies must be mobilized against this problem, and that such organizations as WHO, UNICEF, CIOMS, the International Council for Nurses, and others, should assume a responsibility for jointly and systematically publicizing the magnitude of this problem, its implications for child physical and psychosocial well-being, the factors contributing to it, and the steps that could be taken both internationally and nationally to reduce and eventually control the problem.

The group believed that a new philosophy is called for on the part of such international bodies as the International Monetary Fund, UN groups, bilateral agencies, private foundations and major religious organizations, so as to recognize the priority of this problem. Similarly if gross child abuse of the type being experienced by children in developing countries is to be effectively attacked, national governments, professional bodies and non-governmental groups must also be able to take up this issue.

Specifically Group A recommended that a major thrust be developed by such organizations as WHO, UNICEF, ILO, CIOMS and others, and that a five-year plan of action be jointly developed to organize an advocacy programme that would entail a common message to be communicated aggressively by these organizations, using different educational and communicational mechanisms. These activities should convey the idea that the socially preventable diseases and other health problems, including child labour and child prostitution, currently affecting children who are growing up in poverty and destitution, are the grossest form of child abuse and neglect. These organizations should set targets for the mobilization of economic and technical resources at both international and national levels, and should be in a position to publicly evaluate the progress made at the end of a five-year period. Because the problem is relatively ill-defined in many countries, international groups should seek to stimulate and help with studies to define the form this problem is taking.

Group A also recognized that at the cultural level there is considerable abuse of children as a result of traditional views concerning the status and role of children. As a result of culturally defined practices and attitudes, exploitative child labour and sexually abusive practices appear to be increasing. They are certainly not decreasing, and the number of groups at risk is proliferating as a result of population shifts such as urbanization, and a type of anomic poverty found mainly in new slum and squatter settlements.

Child labour practices that do not permit children to develop to their physical and psychosocial potential and effectively deny them the possibility of participating in a normal social developmental process are widespread in a number of countries.

Child fostering is similarly widespread in many countries and appears to be a form of exploitative child labour that defies any easy definition in terms of magnitude, distribution, and health implications.

In some countries early child marriage and early initiation of sexually related practices are imposing harmful physical and psychological health pressures on, especially female, children.

Excessive corporal punishment, common in some cultural systems and often interpreted as necessary disciplinary action, needs to be addressed to the same extent as the active physical abuse that currently is open to prosecution.

A number of resources can be tapped. Depending upon the level of development of a society, these may range from universities and teacher-training colleges, where components on this issue need to be included in standard curricula. With regard to child labour practices the possible involvement of major international and national labour unions needs to be explored. Similarly women's organizations and parent-teacher groups should be sensitized to the implications for child health of many of the practices that are taken for granted.

The use of mass media and involvement in collaborative public education programmes designed to sensitize the public at all levels need to be emphasized.

Professional associations and non-governmental organizations are in many countries uniquely suited to promoting greater awareness of the ways in which institutionalized, or otherwise socially condoned, practices can and do violate the right to health and development of children.

In many cases it may be necessary to stimulate and support national surveys that demonstrate the physical and psychosocial impact of these practices. Where this is the case, international groups should be active in coordinating and providing technical support to national activities so as to ensure a broad and systematic coverage of the problem.

Specifically the group recommends:

    a) A five-year plan of action that would bring together major inter-governmental and nongovernmental groups in a consolidated programme of advocacy and action, following a common theme, using similar educational documents and materials, and with a common goal

154

and targets. The purpose of this initiative would be to draw the attention of all levels of society to the magnitude of child abuse in the three forms that have been reviewed, namely societal, institutionalized and individual.

b) To achieve this goal the agencies responsible for this conference should prepare and widely disseminate two principal documents:

(i) the report of the conference and the background papers, and

(ii) a booklet prepared along the same clear systematic lines of the guide on child sexual assault, which would describe the forms that child abuse takes, the known magnitude of the problem, its health implications and its social aetiology. The booklet would *not* seek to provide solutions; it is proposed as an informational document to be distributed free of charge to all governmental groups, non-governmental organizations, public communication media, schools, religious bodies, etc.

c) Because much of the work needed is of a social support nature, there should be a careful selection of appropriate non-governmental organizations at international and national levels that are willing and able to take up this issue in a comprehensive way, and these groups should be supported systematically from private and public resources, internationally and nationally.

d) Because many of the forms child abuse takes reflect a growing inability of families to successfully adapt to, and cope with, changing social and ecological conditions, new forms of social support should be promoted and mobilized. These may take the form of community-based nutrition programmes — all designed to help share some of the family responsibilities with respect to child care. With regard to family support action, however, the group noted the unequal distribution of work in families and recommends that ways be explored of encouraging a greater sharing of responsibilities between men and women.

e) The need for innovative action is so acute that models of successful multidisciplinary programmes should be written up and training activities developed around them. If necessary, key programmes in different regions should be taken up by international non-governmental organizations and inter-governmental groups as reference "centres". Resource documents, films, and other media forms should be developed which would take up the issue of child abuse (in its different forms) in clear and systematic ways.

f) The lack of public awareness about child abuse may be the greatest obstacle to dealing with the problem. Television, radio, and the printed media can and should play more of an educational role in this regard. To achieve a consistent message, key organizations should be asked to prepare core messages or programmes that can then be adapted to local media channels.

g) A widespread form of institutionalized maltreatment is the detention of children in so-called correctional centres, where children are exposed to greater physical and sexual abuse than they would be elsewhere. International declarations such as the Tokyo Declaration should be more widely and effectively used. International standards and guidelines should be devised for the design, management and staffing of detention centres involving children, and wherever feasible steps should be taken to introduce guidelines and "rights" governing the "correction" of children.

h) Precocious pregnancy is deleterious to the health and well-being of both the girl (and at times the boy) concerned and her offspring. A responsible recognition by national authorities of the needs for early family planning must be promoted and steps taken to make family life education a well-accepted, positively oriented process that can be incorporated into school programmes.

i) Legislative action is nothing without enforcement mechanisms. Nevertheless, there should be legislative support, and periodic review of legislation and its appropriateness to children's needs.

j) Alternative ways of approaching the problem of child abuse must be sought. The idea of establishing ombudsmen for children's rights should be explored in as many countries as possible.

k) Multidisciplinary approaches to child abuse in its various forms is relatively new. Wherever experiences have been positive, or wherever there is a need to support the initial work being undertaken by countries, exchange programmes should be encouraged so that a critical mass of people can be created sharing common goals and work approaches.

RESOURCES

Reporting	Confidential approach	Review action mechanism	Supportive problem-solving approach
Child			
Adult			
Health professionals			
Teachers			
Neighbours			

Law

The central theme is to have an effective review and action mechanism with a) good liaison with the local legal system, and b) a supportive problem-solving approach. Once this is established, a confidential reporting system could be promoted. This could include reporting by children, adults, teachers, health professionals and neighbours.

Resources available would influence the degree of sophistication that could be achieved. The review action mechanism in an industrialized country would be a comprehensive team, and in non-industrialized rural areas it could be a respected grandmother, for example.

The supportive problem-solving approach would again depend on resources but should be the recommended course of action rather than resorting to a legal adversarial approach.

DISCUSSION

Cantwell: Relating in particular to the detention of children, I have a number of problems — the major problem, apart from certain drafting questions, is that international standards and guidelines do exist or are in the process of formulation. More precisely, at the most recent General Assembly of the United Nations, the Standard Minimum Rules on the Administration of Juvenile Justice were adopted, and at the recent United Nations conference in Milan on the treatment of offenders, a resolution was passed calling for the formulation of standard minimum rules on the protection of juveniles deprived of their freedom; these will indeed cover the concerns which are extremely legitimate concerns expressed in this part of the report. So perhaps the wording could be changed to request that the existing Standard Minimum Rules, which are not binding on governments, they are guidelines, on the administration of justice should be applied, that we urge their application and the formulation of standard minimum rules covering the protection of juveniles deprived of their liberty. One other comment — I strongly suggest that instead of saying "so-called correctional centres" we call them correctional facilities, quite simply. They are not so-called correctional centres: they are correctional facilities where children become especially vulnerable to harmful procedures and practices, including physical and sexual abuse.

GROUP B: Roles of governmental and nongovernmental organizations

Moderator: P. E. Ferrier
Secretary: M. A. Belsey

Child abuse takes many forms and arises from a variety of circumstances. It may be extra-familial or intra-familial, and may be manifest at three levels: global, cultural and individual. Within any particular community the underlying causes, associated pathology and precipitating stresses and events may vary.

Over the last two decades in a number of developed countries attention has been focused upon child abuse as manifested in individuals, i.e., child battering, physical and sexual abuse, and neglect. Mainly, it has received multidisciplinary clinical attention, especially treatment and rehabilitation, including tertiary prevention — the prevention of further progress or effects of the circumstances that gave rise to the problem. To a great extent, child abuse in this form has been seen as a product of deviant behaviour and maltreatment, and often precipitation by, or associated with, familial and social stress. In an effort to better understand the problem and develop approaches to its prevention and treatment, a number of behavioural models have been constructed to describe the relationships and sequence of events leading to child abuse.

Recently the concepts of primary and secondary prevention of child abuse have emerged as broad health and social strategies. Secondary prevention has inherent within it the need to recognize the profile of risk characteristics and circumstances that have a high probability of resulting in child abuse, in order to permit intervention at an individual or community level to ameliorate or prevent the progression of those circumstances. Primary prevention is a much more difficult task; it includes social and health promotion, support for responsible and informed parenthood, and the mobilization of social resources and institutions to ensure healthy family life.

Extra-familial child abuse, particularly that imposed by societies' failings and social inequity, is a far more pervasive phenomenon than the intra-familial variety; it is hidden except in crises, and receives neither adequate attention from the public nor the serious concern of decision-makers. The forms of extra-familial abuse range from child labour, child prostitution, and abandonment to the submitting of whole populations of children to the numbing brutality of war, and the acceptance of violence and different forms of exploitation as societal norms.

Certain common threads of association and causality appear to underlie both extra-familial and intra-familial child abuse: poverty, social inequity, ignorance, racism and unemployment. Intra-familial child abuse, for the most part perpetrated by a parent or other guardian, is associated with social isolation and other kinds of social pathology such as alcoholism and wife battering. There is ample anecdotal evidence that, without timely intervention at the first signs or evidence of child abuse, events progress tragically even to death, permanent physical or mental disability, and repetition of the pattern of abuse in the next generation. For intra-familial physical child abuse the critical ingredients appear to be familial stress and a triggering event.

Although the true magnitude of the problem is unknown, it is known that the broad fabric of social tension, inequity and economic crises contributes directly and indirectly to both intra- and extra-familial child abuse; it seems likely therefore that its incidence will continue and increase unless there is a decisive social and political commitment to broad social and specific coordinated action to deal with it.

Action on child abuse has been forthcoming from the health, social welfare, judicial and other sectors. Many organizations, both governmental and nongovernmental, have accumulated experience and perfected ways of dealing with particular aspects of the problem. What has been lacking, with the exception of a few countries and limited international effort, is to collate and analyse information on these experiences so that it may be widely disseminated and adapted. Also lacking are comprehensive national strategies, and a coordinated global effort to coordinate technical and moral support for national efforts.

The roles and responsibilities of governmental and nongovernmental organizations and agencies, national and international

Child abuse may be examined from three perspectives: organizations; the management of child abuse; and social action and functions. These perspectives may be used as guidelines for promoting, mobilizing and providing technical support to organizations, institutions and agencies at the local, national and international levels.

Organizations and institutions

The range of types of organizations and institutions which are, or should be, directly or indirectly concerned with child abuse may be classed as Non-governmental and Governmental. Non-governmental organizations include professional organizations (such as those of physicians, paediatricians, psychiatrists; nurses; teachers; jurists; and social workers) and community organizations and action groups (organizations sponsored by churches or other religious groups; associations of parents, teachers and children; women and youth groups; trade unions; social welfare/service organizations; consumer groups; and advocacy groups).

Governmental (or public sector) organizations or institutions include ministries of health, social welfare, justice, labour, women, youth, education, etc., and institutions, such as research institutes or councils responsible for health and social research; universities; and mass communication media.

The management of child abuse

The management of "clinical" intra-familial child abuse has evolved with increasing awareness of the nature of the problem and the need of action. It has the following components:

—Creation of social awareness of, and sensitization of the public to, the problem
—Recognition and ascertainment of instances and circumstances of child abuse
—Direct treatment and rehabilitation of the child

159

—Prevention of further damage or deterioration, coupled with continued rehabilitative efforts (tertiary prevention)
—Prevention of other cases by applying the concept of a risk approach
—Provision of special preventive and supportive care in high-risk situations, e.g., premature infants
—Primary prevention, directed at the immediate responsible health and social behaviour to prevent risks from arising, e.g., family-life education and promotion of responsible parenthood, family planning, social support measures and legislation.

Social action and functions

The group agreed on the following broad functions that programmes directed at child abuse should perform; they are equally applicable to the intra-familial and the extra-familial forms of child abuse:

—use of the mass communication media to generate and ensure awareness of the problem
—advocacy of the protection of children's rights
—technical advice, dissemination of information, and support
—direct treatment, rehabilitation and prevention services
—situation-monitoring
—ascertaining need
—formulating policy
—legislative and regulatory action and implementation
—research
—funding and support programmes
—training and standard-setting

Creating awareness

The means whereby different organizations and agencies may promote awareness of the problem of child abuse and neglect may be summarized as follows:

Professional organizations

Physicians/paediatricians	Reliable information to the public, the media, and decision-makers
Jurists, legal sector	Information as to existing and possible legal and regulatory action

Community organizations

Parents, women, trade unions, social welfare, advocacy	Provision of information and community education to the public and to specific groups
Universities/research institutes	Research and dissemination of research findings
Communications/media	Public dissemination of information to promote in a socially responsible way social action and policies

Unless awareness is generated at local, national and international levels, there will not be a critical mass of individuals and organizations to promote and support programmes for the control and elimination of child abuse in its various forms. The establishment of links between the different agencies, organizations and institutions would make it easier for each to exercise its role.

The group recommended that technically and socially involved groups should prepare an awareness-communication strategy. The sharing of experiences with different approaches in creating awareness among national groups and authorities would hasten the achievement of the goal of a more accurately informed and responsive public.

Providing technical advice

Professional organizations of physicians, nurses, jurists, trade unions (national and international organizations) could establish standards and norms of care, monitoring, and formulation of legislation and regulations.

In the discussion on the need for, and use of, technical advice, the group recommended that a focal point for child abuse be designated and appropriately placed within the governmental structure. It would serve the purposes of gathering information, making available technical documentation, advice and materials, and advising national authorities.

Provision of direct services

Direct services involve a large number of disciplines and a variety of agencies, and take on different forms in different developed and developing countries. In such circumstances, unless some agency or organization assumes or is given statutory authority, treatment, rehabilitation and prevention are liable to be neglected or to develop in distorted ways, e.g., purely punitive action, or to be only *ad hoc* and episodic.

No well-organized services can be provided in the absence of explicit or implicit policies and an allocation and acceptance of responsibility and authority. Although there may be no explicit services for child abuse, the broad promotive and preventive approaches inherent in primary health care — healthy and responsible parenthood and child-rearing, supported by community resources — encompass positive action with regard to child abuse. These approaches are applicable in both developed and developing countries, and involve the acceptance of responsibility by, and support to, families, communities and their organizations.

Community organizations, being outside the government structure, have a critical role in establishing and evaluating innovative programmes, drawing together agencies and disciplines. The group recommended that governments and intergovernmental agencies promote and support this role, particularly with regard to the exchange and analysis of experience for the use of concerned national and international organizations.

Various direct service models have been devised — for example, "hot line" crisis management programmes, and multidisciplinary case conference or management groups. Where there are no such direct services, voluntary bodies, with the support of professional organizations, can take an initiative in establishing them. They should of course coordinate and organize their activities in such a way that the community or government, or preferably both, will integrate them in their social services and assure their adequate support.

Conference or management groups for the provision of direct services take various forms but share certain features. The model that provides treatment, rehabilitation and tertiary prevention needs to be well staffed with skilled people and is not immediately applicable to many developing countries.

The group recommended that priority consideration be given to primary prevention of child abuse in its various manifestations, as part of promotive and preventive child health and care, within the context of primary health care. Primary prevention includes means whereby families, communities and their organizations acquire knowledge and skills; training of staff in the necessary educational skills; and the provision of coordinated supportive services and care by the health, social, legal and other sectors, appropriate to a country's resources and policies.

The group drew attention to existing United Nations and other international instruments and standards relating to the protection and promotion of the rights and well-being of young persons; these include the Declaration on the Rights of the Child, in particular Article 9, relating to child abuse and neglect; the United Nations Standard Minimum Rules for Juvenile Justice; and the Draft Convention on the Rights of the Child. These could in due course provide an impetus for national action.

RECOMMENDATIONS

There should be technical interdisciplinary coordination at regional and international levels, among the United Nations Organization and its specialized agencies and other intergovernmental bodies, and in the nongovernmental sphere, as well as between those two sectors. One function of such coordination would be to provide a channel for the exchange of information and experience between governmental and nongovernmental agencies with a view to fostering progress in responding to the problem of child abuse, neglect and exploitation.

Noting that the role of a child within a family may be a reflection of the role of the family and the child in society, the group recommended that each country should designate a focus for the promotion and protection of children's rights, needs and interests.

WHO and other interested organizations, including nongovernmental organizations, should consider preparing a survey of policy, law and practice relating to the prevention and control of child abuse and neglect in selected developed and developing countries. National contributions would reflect government policies and institutional frameworks as well as the viewpoints of voluntary bodies with regard to key problems and possible solutions, and would be structured according to a commonly-agreed format to facilitate the sharing of national experiences.

WHO should establish a team or task force, representing various countries and disciplines, which could respond to requests for technical cooperation from countries wishing to review policy, or to develop a new policy, on combating child abuse and neglect.

Noting that the magnitude and effects of the problem of child abuse and neglect (intra- and extra-familial) are insufficiently known and acknowledged, and, consequently, that action to prevent, discover and treat child abuse and neglect is often uncoordinated and hence not fully effective, the group recommended that, where appropriate, governmental authorities should endeavour to formulate national policy on the subject of child abuse and neglect, which would, *inter alia,* specify the roles of governmental and nongovernmental organizations and provide for the designation and coordination of resources and services.

GROUP C: Gaps in knowledge

Moderator: R. Krugman
Secretary: P. M. Shah

Most countries have very little or no information about the definition of child abuse and neglect. Obviously, definitions will vary according to social norms of accepted behaviour and child-rearing, and a country's economic development and socio-political system.

The definition of child abuse and neglect should take account of the child's views of what constitutes abuse. In other words, any intended or unintended act or omission by an adult, society or country which adversely affects the child's health, physical growth and psychosocial development should be considered as abuse or neglect — even if the child does not regard it as abuse or neglect, and, conversely, a child may justifiably feel abused even though adults do not recognize a particular form of abuse as such.

Other forms of abuse found in society include, but are not limited to: exploitative child labour, vagrancy or homelessness involving children, child prostitution, and the effects on children of war, including their involvement as child combatants.

Sexual abuse of the child is being discussed and investigated in many countries. Legal and medical definitions of sexual abuse differ. Many of the disclosures of sexual abuse at present come from adolescents, but younger children when questioned also relate instances of abuse. Children's reports of being sexually abused are almost always true. In general, however, sexual abuse of children remains hidden, owing to familial and societal denial and taboos. Moreover, laws that affect children, which are made by adults, need to be balanced by consideration of the child's welfare and by provisions to ensure children's rights of control over their own bodies.

In developed countries, information about child abuse is often collected by organized official reporting systems. Lay reporting and informal surveys are other means of obtaining information. Methods of collecting information in developing countries need to evolve locally, keeping in mind that poor record-keeping and high rates of illiteracy are prevalent.

The use of home-visiting by staff of voluntary organizations or other lay people needs to be explored. It may be associated with professional services. Community leaders, elders and religious leaders can be involved in both information-gathering and intervention.

Lack of opportunity for education should be considered as neglect, and information is needed on ways of providing education to the large numbers of children who are deprived of it.

There is a special need to modify the content and the methods of education of such deprived children if it is to accomplish anything worthwhile.

Packaged educational material might be helpful in sensitizing children to aspects of child abuse. Empirical data are required for the preparation and use of such material for school-age children.

164

Intra-familial child neglect occurs with regard to diet and nutrition. In many societies in developing countries girls are neglected when food is being served as compared with boys, and children are fed only after the adults have eaten.

Gaps in knowledge about child abuse and neglect are enormous and too numerous to list. The conference agreed on a recommendation of an *approach* that any country or organization could use to deal with the problem.

Recommendation

The problem of child abuse and neglect requires a focal point in government with responsibility for children's programmes.

The focal point should:

(1) Collect information (by formal and informal means) about the forms and extent of the problem
(2) Determine its magnitude
(3) Set priorities for dealing with it
(4) Determine roles for those who will work on the problem (e.g., the child, the family, professionals, and governmental and nongovernmental agencies)
(5) Increase awareness of the problem among both the general public and professionals
(6) Devise approaches to solving the problem
    a) universal vs. at-risk populations (e.g., individuals — adolescent parents; groups — migrants; areas — urban slums)
    b) develop a system for discovery, referral and treatment of "victims" and "offenders"
    c) develop preventive programmes involving the health system, educational systems (formal and informal), the work-place, and wherever children are found
    d) develop adult/child education programmes (e.g., on parental functioning, family life, child abuse, children's rights)
(7) Professional and paraprofessional workers
(8) Develop evaluation and research methods to monitor progress or introduce changes

Some requirements for implementation of the above recommendation include, but are not limited to:

(1) Designation of a key, committed body with adequate resources and authority
(2) Adequate training of individuals for the task. This should include basic curriculum, continuing consultation, continuing education, and monitoring of competence
(3) A multidisciplinary approach
(4) Support-systems for workers
(5) Involvement of voluntary, lay, "self help" or other community groups.

GENERAL DISCUSSION

Shamma': I would just emphasize one point: as regards probably all areas of child abuse except child abuse secondary to war, there is a great deal that people in various fields — health, legal, social — can do. The problem as regards children in war is that such groups on their own do not determine whether a war is going to take place, and for years wars have taken place in spite of organizations, national and international, that have worked towards the end of war and world-wide disarmament. I suggest one thing, a single specific act, that people in the health field can do, and that might help increase attention and sensitivity to the problem of children in war, and that is to include death from war and war-related injuries in the International Classification of Diseases. This would probably be the greatest achievement possible in the field of child abuse. I should think it unfortunate if from this conference there would not be a specific recommendation on that point.

Gellhorn: Thank you very much, Dr Shamma'. It seems very appropriate to raise this here, and with Dr Bettex here it is my guess that there is a possibility, at any rate, that the paediatric surgeons might be willing to consider this issue of war-related, surgical traumatic injuries to children not only in the preparation of ICD-10 but also in the development of a nomenclature of diseases, in which CIOMS is involved — it would be a very powerful way of calling attention to the problem. Perhaps Dr Bettex would be willing to give this some consideration. It is my impression that the paucity of comments is related to the fact that it is very difficult to absorb these brief summaries of the work of the working groups without having a document before us, and also not having had the opportunity — even if the document were before us — to read it and think about the implications. I can say, from the standpoint of CIOMS, that the proceedings of this conference will be published as rapidly as possible, and that the publication will be widely distributed. Now, as a lay participant in the conference I shall try to summarize what it has meant to me, and then we could perhaps hear from others what it has meant to them. I am enormously impressed that once again we have a widely interdisciplinary group of people who have been brought together to consider a very significant subject, and it seems to me that this reflects not only the importance of the problem but also a way of approaching problems. Today, it is increasingly less pertinent for individual groups to attempt to solve problems that have broad implications, and the fact that we have come together from so many different backgrounds, of training and experience, to say nothing of countries, has been very impressive. I also leave this conference with a far broader conception of the issues of child abuse and neglect than I had when I came. Yesterday's presentations emphasized not only the physical abuse of children, with which we are all familiar, but also the abuse and neglect associated with the street children or vagrant children, those who have suffered from national and international policies that have placed greater priorities on allocating resources for armaments than for food. Dr Shamma''s very compelling comments from her experience in Lebanon broadened my concept considerably. Also, I now understand better the qualitative and quantitative differences in child abuse and neglect between the developing and developed countries.

An important distinction seems to be that in the industrialized countries a great deal of attention is given to curative efforts as well as to prevention but the developing countries have so few resources and the problem is so great that they must give attention to prevention. I am enormously grateful to all the participants here for what I have learned. Our group discussions have been extraordinarily fruitful both as a means of communication among us and for the depth that they achieved. I conclude then, finally, with the question, which is more difficult — to have space-walkers orbiting the earth at 27,000 miles an hour and building a tower like a tinker toy, or to build decent housing in the world's barrios and slums; to perfect an intercontinental missile which can destroy vast countries in seven minutes rather than the present 30 minutes, or to develop personnel to educate comprehensively families, health professionals, justice officials, all those who are concerned with the prevention and cure of child abuse and neglect? All of these possibilities are within our resources. Each depends on decision and will. We hope that the imagination which is unlocked for armaments in outer space may be unlocked for grace and beauty in the daily lives of children. Our economy needs it and I believe that our society will perish without it. And, it seems to me that, although, as Dr Shamma' indicated, we are not in a position to control the declarations of war, we can make some contribution to the future of children throughout the world through our efforts in our countries, our communities, with our various associations, if we keep in mind the allocation and the misallocation of resources.

Krugman: Mr Chairman, yours are eloquent words. I would add only one thing — to reiterate what I said the first day about one at a time — and that is that we are dealing with complex problems; wherever and however and whatever the problems are that we are dealing with they are enormous. It is also clear that those who care for children, in all senses of the word 'care', do so as a fairly significant minority group among those who care for the rest of the humans in the world. As such it is more difficult work. However, complex problems don't have simple solutions — they have numerous solutions, many many different approaches, and for me it was refreshing to hear about different approaches and different ideas, because we sometimes hope that our way will be the way to solve the world's problems, when the reality is that there have to be numerous approaches to them, and we all need to support one another in all of these approaches whatever they are, whether they seem tangential to what we are doing or seem right on target. The other thing that I think gatherings like this do is to refresh the brain and rekindle the flame for those who are spending their lives day by day trudging around in the trenches, working with very difficult problems of very maltreated children, very difficult families in very difficult environments. For that experience, I thank the organizing group and others for inviting me and all of you for giving me the opportunity to work a little better, I hope, over the next six months or year or so, before I fade and need another one of these.

Belsey: Some of my colleagues have heard me quote from Oliver Wendell Holmes who, some 75 or 80 years ago, stated "it is the practice of knowledge to speak, it is the privilege of wisdom to listen". It characterizes the spirit and the methodology of this conference, from which we have all learned so much. Many of us have listened very attentively in this meeting. We have heard the voices of those who are not here, the voices of the battered child, the voices that are stilled or muffled by gunfire, hunger, or any of the other socially abusive experiences which they suffer every day. Perhaps the other important lesson from this conference is that we are not alone — by coming together and being patient and listening to one another, by exchanging experiences, by being open and realizing that none of our separate experiences may be the complete answer, and that a complementary answer may be found half way around the world, or even next door, we have learned that we are not alone. It has also, I think, reinforced the approach and process of listening, not only to one another as professionals but also to communities, and to people, being patient and hearing them out. I should like with those words, on behalf of my colleagues in WHO, to thank the participants for continuing my in-service education, by giving me a richness of experience and insight that we have the privilege to carry to other countries. All of you have made outstanding contributions in the discussions and in the papers, and I look forward to both working with and continuing with Dr Bankowski, in realizing the rapid publication of the proceedings. I take the opportunity to thank particularly Dr Bettex for his persistence in pursuing with interest and urgency the problem of battered children and child abuse and seeing the implementation of an outstanding conference here in Berne, with truly outstanding facilities and support from both Dr Kehrer and Dr Slongo. I thank also my fellow WHO staff members for their support in assisting in the organization of this meeting. Finally, I should like to state that CIOMS has a long history of collaboration and a vital role in the field of health and social and political issues relevant to health globally. I would particularly thank Dr Bankowski for giving us the opportunity to work with CIOMS in seeing through a conference which I think will be a milestone in redirecting and reorienting our thinking, and perhaps the world's thinking, on what constitutes an abused and neglected child, and how to stop such abuse and neglect.

CLOSING OF CONFERENCE
Murillo Belchior

Before closing the meeting, I would like to express, on behalf of the CIOMS, our sincere appreciation and high recognition of the Local Organizing Committee from Berne, especially Professor M.C. Bettex, Dr B. Kehrer and Dr T. Slongo, who organized this conference in a most professional manner and with a pleasant friendly atmosphere. As I mentioned a couple of days ago, Professor Bettex can be fully satisfied that his idea of six or so years ago has finally materialized into a productive, international forum on an important topic.

It is my pleasure once again to thank very much our colleagues from the World Health Organization, particularly Dr A. Petros-Barvazian, Dr Belsey, Dr Carballo and Dr Shah, whose technical know-how and experience were invaluable in the preparation of the conference and the carrying out of its deliberations.

I would like to underline that this conference became a reality thanks to the substantial financial support received from the Max and Elsa Beer-Brawand Fund, the Swiss Academy of Medical Sciences, the Swiss National Fund and Migros Enterprise.

It is a real pleasure for me to express our thanks to the former President of CIOMS, Alfred Gellhorn, whose leadership as a Chairman of this conference was, as usual, on an extremely high level, conducting us all with ease through the deliberations.

It must not be forgotten to mention that we are all very grateful to all those persons — behind the scenes — involved in the preparations and technical arrangements. Though they are not always seen during the conference, their presence was indispensable.

I cannot end these few words without speaking of Dr Bankowski and Miss Amsler, whose hard work, dedication and efficiency greatly contributed to the success of this conference.

LIST OF PARTICIPANTS

ABELIN, T. Institute of Social and Preventive Medicine, University of Berne, Berne, Switzerland

ADADEVOH, B.K. Vice-President, Council for International Organizations of Medical Sciences, Ebute-Metta, Nigeria

ADEKUNLE, O. Confederation of African Medical Associations and Societies, Ibadan, Nigeria

AKHMISSE, M. Ministry of Public Health, Casablanca, Morocco

ALTHAUS, J. Klinik für Pädiatrie, Medical University of Lübeck, Lübeck, Federal Republic of Germany

BANKOWSKI, Z. Executive Secretary, Council for International Organizations of Medical Sciences, Geneva, Switzerland

BARBOSA, A. Children's Protection Service, Ministry of Justice, Lisbon, Portugal

BARRON, P. Department of Health, Dublin, Ireland

BAY, M. Maternité, Centre hospitalier universitaire vaudois, Lausanne, Switzerland

BELCHIOR, M. President, Council for International Organizations of Medical Sciences, Rio de Janeiro, Brazil

BELL, B. Faculty of Community Medicine & Social Studies, Newcastle-upon-Tyne Polytechnic, Newcastle-upon-Tyne, England

BELSEY, M. Maternal and Child Health Unit, W.H.O., Geneva, Switzerland

BETTEX, M. World Federation of Associations of Pediatric Surgeons; Chirurgische Universitäts-Kinderklinik, Berne, Switzerland

BETTEX-GALLAND, M. Chirurgische Universitäts-Kinderklinik, Berne, Switzerland

BLAND, J. Division of Public Information and Education for Health, W.H.O., Geneva, Switzerland

BOEHLEN, M. National Council of Women in Switzerland, Zürich, Switzerland

BOICHIS, H. Sackler Faculty of Medicine, Tel-Aviv University, Tel-Aviv, Israel

BRÄGGER C. Kinderspital Zürich, Eleonorenstiftung Universitäts-Kinderklinik, Zürich, Switzerland

BROWNE, K.D. International Society for the Study of Behavioural Development, Surrey, England

BRUCE, F. International Catholic Child Bureau, Geneva, Switzerland

CAFFO, E. University of Modena, Bologna, Italy

CANTWELL, N. Defence for Children International, Geneva, Switzerland

CARBALLO, M. Maternal and Child Health Unit, W.H.O., Geneva, Switzerland

CARMICHAEL, A. Royal Children's Hospital, Parkville, Victoria, Australia

CLARA, R. Universitaire Instelling Antwerpen, Wilrijk, Belgium

COTTIER, E. Ministère public du canton de Vaud, Lausanne, Switzerland

COURVOISIER, B. Swiss Academy of Medical Sciences, Geneva, Switzerland

de DARDEL, T. Service de Protection de la Jeunesse, Lausanne, Switzerland

DIAZ, R. United Nations Children Fund (UNICEF), Eastern and Southern Africa Regional Office, Nairobi, Kenya

DOEK, J. International Society for the Prevention of Child Abuse and Neglect; Vrije Universiteit, Amsterdam, Netherlands

DOGRAMACI, I. International Pediatric Association, Paris, France

DUNNING, M. Department of Health and Social Security, London, England

EHRENSPERGER, J. Kinderspital Wildermeth, Biel, Switzerland

ELLIOTT, M. Child Assault Prevention Programme, London, England

ELY, B. Department of Health and Social Security, London, England

ENNEW, J. Cambridge Institute for the Study of Industrial Societies, Kings College, Cambridge, England

ESTERMANN-JANSEN, C. Schweitz., Stiftung MPB, Berne, Switzerland

EUGENE-DAHIN, B. Institut de Médecine Légale, Liège, Belgium

FARBER, J. President-elect, World Medical Association, Brussels, Belgium

FARSANG, C. Federation of Hungarian Medical Societies, Budapest, Hungary

FERRIER, P.E. Department of Paediatrics and Genetics, University of Geneva, Geneva, Switzerland

FLORIS, C. Assistance sociale, Geneva, Switzerland

FLUSS, S.S. Health Legislation Unit, W.H.O., Geneva, Switzerland

FORSTER, Ch. University Children's Hospital, Münich, Federal Republic of Germany

GAILLARD, R. International Council of Women, Lausanne, Switzerland

GELLHORN, A. Council for International Organizations of Medical Sciences; New York State Department of Health, Albany, New York, U.S.A.

GEORGES, T. College of Medicine, Howard University, Washington, D.C., U.S.A.

GHOBRIAL, C.F. Ministry of Health, Cairo, Egypt

GILL, D. International Federation of Surgical Colleges, Dublin, Ireland

GIORDANA, M. Holy See, Apostolic Nunciature, Berne, Switzerland

GNEHM, H. University Children's Hospital, Zürich, Switzerland

GOERMER, P. Ministère public du canton de Vaud, Lausanne, Switzerland

GOODWIN, S. Home Visitors Association, United Kingdom

HACHEN, H.J. International Rehabilitation Medicine Association, Geneva, Switzerland

HANIMANN, B. Kinderchirurgische Klinik Kinderspital, St. Gallen, Switzerland

HAY, I.T. Medunsa University & Department of Health, Medunsa, Republic of South Africa

HEICK, C. Kinderspital Zürich, Eleonorenstiftung Universitäts-Kinderklinik, Zürich, Switzerland

HERZOG, J. Sozialversicherung, Berne, Switzerland

HIRNSPERGER, G. Verein Arbeitsgemeinshcaft gegen Kindermissbrauch, Innsbruck, Austria

HÖLLWARTH, M. Universitäts-Klinik für Kinderchirurgie, Graz, Austria

HORDE, G. Mission de Coopération française, Djibouti

HURNI-CAILLE, L. Schweizerischer Kinderschutzbund, Berne, Switzerland

JANSSENS, P.G. Comité des Académies royales de Médecine, 'S Gravenwezel, Belgium

JUNOD, B. Chirurgische Universitäts-Kinderklinik, Berne, Switzerland

KANTORIK, W. Swiss Group against "Legal Kidnapping" Abduction of Children, Biel, Switzerland

KEHRER, B. Chirurgische Universitäts-Kinderklinik, Berne, Switzerland

KIRCHGASSLER, K. University of Giessen, Giessen, Federal Republic of Germany

KOENEN, I. Köln, Federal Republic of Germany

KOHLER, P. Cantonal Ministry of Education, Berne, Switzerland

KÖNIG, E.R. International Society of Audiology, Basel, Switzerland

KRUGMAN, R.D. C. Henry Kempe National Center for the Prevention and Treatment of Child Abuse and Neglect, Denver, Colorado, U.S.A.

LAMPING-GOOS, M.D. Chief Medical Office of Mental Health, Leidschendam, Netherlands

LAMPING-GOOS, P. Gynaecologist, Schalkmaar, Netherlands

LANDY, R. Division of Public Information and Education for Health, W.H.O., Geneva, Switzerland

LEHMANN, P. International Sociological Association, Lausanne, Switzerland

LENKO, H.L. University of Tampere, Department of Clinical Sciences, Tampere, Finland

LESNIK OBERSTEIN, M. Free University of Amsterdam, Amsterdam, Netherlands

LOBO FERNANDES, M.J. Instituto de Apoio à Criança, Lisbon, Portugal

MALENGA, G. W.H.O. Regional Office for Africa, Kilongwe, Malawi

MARTIN, J.F. Swiss Society for Social and Preventive Medicine, Lausanne, Switzerland

MASSON, O. Service Médico-pédagogique vaudois, Service universitaire de Psychiatrie de l'Enfant et de l'Adolescent, Lausanne, Switzerland

MICHEL, P. Groupe de travail pour la prévention des mauvais traitements envers les enfants, Payerne, Switzerland

MORROW, H. International Council of Nurses, Geneva, Switzerland

MOTZEL, C. Medical Women's International Association, Cologne, Federal Republic of Germany

MÖWINCKEL, C. Antwerp Confidential Doctor Centre, University of Antwerp, Antwerp, Belgium

MULLIS, P. Kinderspital, Kinderchirurgische Abteilung, Luzern, Switzerland

MUSIL, E. International Federation for Hygiene, Preventive and Social Medicine, Vienna, Austria

NAIDU, U.S. Tata Institute for Social Sciences, Bombay, India

NASSAUER, A. Universitäts-Kinderklinik, Frankfurt-am-Main, Federal Republic of Germany

NG, T.K.-W. Office of Occupational Health, W.H.O., Geneva, Switzerland

NIEDERLAND, R.T. Czechoslovak Medical Society, Bratislava, Czechoslovakia

OBIKEZE, D.S. Department of Sociology/Anthropology, University of Nigeria, Nsukka-Anambra State, Nigeria

OLATUNBOSUN, D. University of Ibadan, Ibadan, Nigeria

ONYANGO, P. University of Nairobi, Department of Sociology, Nairobi, Kenya

OSELKA, G. Federal Council of Medicine, Sao Paulo, Brazil

OWEN, M. Barrister-at-Law, London, England

PAULI, H.G. Institute for Research in Education and Evaluation, Faculty of Medicine, University of Berne, Berne, Switzerland

PETROS-BARVAZIAN, A. Division of Family Health, W.H.O., Geneva, Switzerland

PINTAUD, C. Sandoz Ltd., Basel, Switzerland

RAPOPORT, S.M. Council for Coordination of the Medical-Scientific Societies of the German Democratic Republic, Berlin, German Democratic Republic

REYES ROMERO, F. Ministry of Health, Bogota, Colombia

RIEDERER, S. Pro Juventute, Zürich, Switzerland

ROMANOFF, A. International Agency for Research on Cancer, Lyon, France

ROOS, B. Federal Office of Public Health, Berne, Switzerland

RUEGG, F. International Catholic Child Bureau, Geneva, Switzerland

SCHMID, P.K. Holy See, Apostolic Nunciature, Berne, Switzerland

SEIGE, K. International Society of Internal Medicine, Halle/S, German Democratic Republic

SHADAM, J. Maternal and Child Health Clinic (WHO), Kabul, Afghanistan

SHAH, P.M. Maternal and Child Health Unit, W.H.O., Geneva, Switzerland

SHAMMA', A. Barbir Hospital, Beirut, Lebanon

SHEHATA, M. General Organization of Teaching Hospitals and Institutes, Cairo, Egypt

SLONGO, T. Chirurgische Universitäts-Kinderklinik, Berne, Switzerland

SOMMER, B. Danish International Development Agency (DANIDA), Copenhagen, Denmark

von STEIGER, A. Physiotherapist, Berne, Switzerland

STUCKI, H-R.R. Jugendpsychiatrie, Berne, Switzerland

STURM, H. Wiener-Pflege u. Adoptiveltern-Verein, Vienna, Austria

THYANGATHYANGA, D. W.H.O. Regional Office for Africa, Lilongwe, Malawi

TSCHÄPPELER, H. International Society of Radiology, Berne, Switzerland

UNTERDORFER, H. Institut für gerichtliche Medizin der Universität, Innsbruck, Austria

VELLA, A. Bulleen 3105, Victoria, Australia

VESTERDAL, J. Department of Paediatrics, Glostrup Hospital, Glostrup, Denmark

VEYER, C. Wiener-Pflege und Adoptiveltern-Verein, Vienna, Austria

VICCICA, A.D. United Nations, Crime Prevention and Criminal Justice Branch, Vienna, Austria

VILARDELL, F. Vice-President, Council for International Organizations of Medical Sciences; World Organization of Gastroenterology, Barcelona, Spain

WATTS, F. Psychiatrist, Warren, Michigan, U.S.A.

WERRO, M. Swiss Group against "Legal Kidnapping" Abduction of Children, Biel, Switzerland

WIMMERSBERGER, A. Kinderspital Zürich, Eleonorenstiftung Universitäts-Kinderklinik, Zürich, Switzerland

WOLTERS, W. University Hospital for Children and Adolescents, Utrecht, Netherlands

ZÖCHLING, M. Verein Arbeitsgemeinschaft gegen Kindermissbrauch, Innsbruck, Austria

ZUPPINGER, K. Medizinische Kinderpoliklinik, Inselspital, Berne, Switzerland